Dementia and
Alzheimer Caregiver's
Survival Guide

Ogechi Hope, DrPH, MSN, RN

ISBN

Hardcover: 978-1-967616-50-3

Paperback: 978-1-967616-51-0

Acknowledgment

I would like to thank my friends and family for their love and support and their understanding through this time. I am also thankful to the caregivers who inspired me to write this book, your dedication to your loved ones is immeasurable. To my colleagues in the healthcare field, thank you for your devotion to improving the lives of those affected by Dementia and Alzheimer's disease.

I hope that this guide provides caregivers with the practical tools and emotional support they need to navigate their journey with strength, hope, and a sense of community. My mission is to empower you, and I am very grateful for this opportunity to share this resource with you.

About the Author

The author brings expertise and genuine compassion to her work with Dementia and Alzheimer's caregivers. With a Doctorate in Public Health and extensive experience as a Registered Nurse and Certified Case Manager, Dr. Hope has dedicated her career to navigating the complexities of chronic illness and empowering families within the healthcare system. Her years of managing care for individuals with chronic conditions have given her unique insights into the challenges patients and their caregivers face.

Beyond her professional qualifications, she understands caregiving's profound emotional and practical demands. She has witnessed firsthand the strength and resilience of families facing the challenges of Alzheimer's disease.

The author's purpose in writing this book is to support the caregiving experience by offering practical guidance and a beacon of hope and strength. She empowers caregivers with the knowledge to ease the weight of loneliness, exhaustion, and overwhelm while nurturing a sense of community and shared understanding in managing care and disease.

Her comprehensive approach, combined with her extensive public health knowledge and practical case management experience, makes her an invaluable resource for those navigating the complexities of Dementia and Alzheimer's care. Her work is a testament to her commitment to empowering caregivers and providing them with the tools and support necessary to provide compassionate and effective care.

Table of Contents

Acknowledgment I

About The Author II

Dedication V

Disclaimer... VI

Foreword.. VII

Part Ii: *Golden Years, Golden Care* 1

Chapter 1: The Silvering World............................ 3

Chapter 2: What Do Your Elderly Loved Ones Or Patients Need And Want? 15

Chapter 3: The Physical Needs Are Important! 31

Part Ii: *Love, Loss, And Dementia* 57

Chapter 4: Demystifying Dementia.......................... 59

Chapter 5: Preparing For Diagnosis 77

Chapter 6: The Misdiagnosis Challenge 91

Chapter 7: The Road Ahead................................. 103

Chapter 8: Managing Behavioral Changes..................... 123

Part Iii: *Senior Care Options*............................. 135

Chapter 9: Aging Well At Home............................. 137

Chapter 10: Making The Move To Assisted Living.......... 151

Chapter 11: When Medical Needs Increase..................... 163

Part Iv: *Thriving In Later Life*.......................... 177

Chapter 12: Staying Active, Staying Independent............. 179

Chapter 13: The Importance Of Social Engagement In Later Life.. 187

Part V: *Supporting The Supporters* 197

Chapter 14: Before You Can Give, Take Care................... 199

Chapter 15: United In Caring.. 214

Part Vi: *Legal And Financial Essentials* 225

Chapter 16: A Legal Framework For Elder Care............... 227

Chapter 17: Planning For The Financial Realities 240

Dedication

This book is dedicated to those who provide compassionate care, ensuring dignity and connection for individuals living with Dementia and Alzheimer's. May this book offer you tools to navigate this journey with grace.

Disclaimer

This book is for informational and educational purposes only. It is not a substitute for professional medical, legal, or psychological advice.

The author and publisher disclaim any liability for loss, injury, or damage resulting from the use of information contained in this book. All caregiving decisions should be made in consultation with appropriate professionals and aligned with the individual's specific needs.

Names and identifying details in case examples may have been changed to protect privacy. Any resemblance to actual persons, living or deceased, is purely coincidental unless otherwise stated.

Foreword

I have the privilege of being asked to write the *Foreword* to this book. As a physician who has practiced and worked with patients with Dementia and Alzheimer's disease, I recommend it.

I have known Dr. Ogechi Hope for more than a decade. She is a seasoned Registered Nurse, Certified Case Manager, and Doctor of Public Health with years of hands-on experience supporting families and managing chronic illnesses. She brings clarity, strength, and understanding to one of the most demanding roles a person can take on.

This book should guide Caregivers in working with individuals affected by Alzheimer's disease and other forms of dementia. It seeks to empower the Caregiver with the tools needed to manage the short—and long-term demands of the job, hence the title, which refers to it as a survival guide. The author states that to care for others, you must first learn to care for yourself. This book offers the support, guidance, and strength needed to walk this path with confidence and compassion.

This book guides Caregivers in managing the emotional, financial, legal, and practical challenges that may arise during their work. It also draws attention to the resources available to them for support and information, offering help whenever needed. Additionally, self-care techniques for better physical and emotional well-being are included.

This is a must-read book for Caregivers of this group of individuals. The author's expertise in this field is one reason this well-researched book should be a companion for people in this line of work. The author is passionate about her work and motivated by her desire to increase the Caregivers' efficiency by also caring for themselves.

I have had the honor of writing this Foreword, not just because I am familiar with the writer but also because I have managed these individuals and know the job's demands.

The book offers valuable insight to Caregivers on how to care for themselves while fulfilling their duties

By

Dr. Chizom Umunna, MBBS

Part I:
Golden Years, Golden Care

Chapter 1: The Silvering World

Everyone has a tale to tell. The story of aging is one that unites us. From the youngest to the oldest, we are all on this journey together. While the pace and hurdles of aging vary, it's a path that everyone steps on.

As we grow older, our bodies and minds undergo changes. The energy of youth gradually transforms into a slower pace. When you were a child, can you recall not being weary from running around all day? Now, when you have to bend over to tie your shoelaces, you might grunt a little! However, those who are older than us are dealing with far more issues than we are right now.

Aging is a complex experience that involves a blend of various changes that happen over time. Human bodies are like machines, and with age, they wear down. We might experience slower reflexes, weaker muscles, and changes in our senses like sight and hearing. This can impact our mobility and how we interact with the world.

How we think and feel can also shift as we age. We might become more reflective, think more about the past, or experience new emotions. There can also be changes in memory and cognitive function.

It's important to that the pace and experience of these changes vary greatly from person to person. It's a complex interplay between the genes, lifestyle choices, and environment.

How the World's Population is Aging

Globally, there are major shifts occurring in the age makeup within our populations. Because our societies were relatively young for most of human history, this transition is exceptional. However, there are two main causes for the recent changes. First of all, better healthcare and overall better living conditions in modern times have helped. Second, there are fewer babies being born, so there are fewer young people compared to older people. This means the average age of the population is going up. While people moving from one place to another (migration) can also affect these numbers, it's not as important as the other two reasons.

The world's population has exploded in the last 50 years. In 1950, there were only 2.5 billion people on Earth. Now, there are over 7 billion of us! And it's not stopping there. According to research,[1] we could reach 9 billion by 2050 and a staggering 11 billion by almost the end of the century.

While the overall population is booming, there's an interesting shift happening. The number of young people (aged 0-14) isn't growing as fast as it used to. At the same time, the number of working-age adults (15-59) has been climbing steadily, especially in poorer countries. However, in richer nations, the percentage of people in this age group is expected to shrink by about half by 2100.

The number of older people is skyrocketing. This is a completely new situation in human history. People aged 60

---

[1] Bloom, D. E., & Luca, D. L. (2016). The Global Demography of Aging: Facts, explanations, future. *SSRN Electronic Journal, Discussion Paper No. 10163.* https://doi.org/10.2139/ssrn.2834213

and over are growing faster than ever before. In 1950, there were only 200 million of them. Today, that number is a huge 760 million! And it's going to keep climbing. By 2050, there could be 2 billion older people, and by 2100, a mind-boggling 3 billion!

Those aged 80 and over have seen a dramatic increase. In 1950, there were only 14 million of them, but by 2015, that number had jumped to 108 million. It is predicted that this number could reach a staggering 900 million by 2100.

This rapid aging has major consequences. People in their 80s and beyond often face serious health issues that require expensive care. This puts a huge strain on our societies and governments. With fewer young people working and more older people needing support, there could be problems with pensions, healthcare, and the economy. Additionally, we don't fully understand the quality of life for these growing numbers of elderly people.

The challenges are momentous. Where will all these older people live? How will we care for them? Some experts worry that a rapidly aging population could slow down economic growth. It's a complex issue that affects people, families, and governments alike.

But there's hope. History has shown us that humans are adaptable. We can find new ways to deal with these challenges. Technology, new laws, and changes in how we work and live can help. For example, we might need to rethink retirement age, make workplaces more family-friendly, improve healthcare, invest in education, and encourage people to save more for their future. By working together, we can turn these challenges into opportunities.

Genetics and Aging

A key aspect in the rate at which the body ages is genetics. You may have noticed that while some people age slowly, others experience the effects of aging a little faster. That's due to our genetic blueprint.

Special instructions to make proteins that repair and protect our DNA are encoded in our genes. The twist is that it can completely alter the game if you have any genetic variances in those instructions. As the years pass, your body may get better or worse at maintaining optimal health. All in all, a person's ability to age gracefully is influenced by their genes.

Our genes also influence how our bodies handle our daily lives. What we eat, how much we exercise, and even the environment we're in can be affected by our genetic makeup. Some people are blessed to have genes that help them thrive on a healthy lifestyle, while others might find it a bit harder. For example, our genes can determine how well our bodies process food and fight inflammation, both of which are linked to general health and how long we live.

Genetics also increase the risk of certain age-related diseases. If a person has a family history of Alzheimer's, heart disease, or certain cancers, it might be due to genetic factors.

But genes aren't the whole story. Lifestyle matters a lot, too. What you eat, how much you exercise, and how you handle stress can all affect how your genes work. This is called epigenetics. Basically, your lifestyle can 'turn on' or 'turn off' certain genes. So, while your genes set the stage, your lifestyle also plays a major role.

Cellular Aging

Our bodies age at the cellular level. This process, called cellular aging or senescence, is where the story of aging unfolds. Over time, our cells become less efficient and can't replicate as well as they used to.

Telomeres are protective caps at the ends of our chromosomes. With each cell division, these caps get shorter. When they become too short, cells can no longer divide and start to age. This is called cellular senescence and contributes to slow wound healing and decreased tissue repair.

Telomere length acts as a cell's biological clock. Longer telomeres mean the cell is young, while shorter telomeres indicate an older cell. Shorter telomeres are linked to age-related diseases like heart disease, cancer, and brain problems.

Telomerase is an enzyme that can extend telomeres, preventing them from getting shorter. It is active in cells that need to divide often, like stem cells. While increasing telomerase activity might slow aging and extend cell life, too much can cause cancer by making cells grow uncontrollably.

In summary, telomeres help control how cells age. Their length is influenced by genetics, environment, and lifestyle. Scientists are still studying telomeres to understand aging better and find ways to help us age more healthily. There's still a lot to learn about this.

Common Changes in An Aging Body

Let's take a closer look into the topic of aging and examine some of the typical physical and health changes that frequently accompany the process. Gaining insight and understanding into these areas can help you in the aging process for yourself and the people you care for.

Bones and Muscles

Our bones naturally become less dense as we age, making them more prone to fractures. At the same time, our muscles can lose strength and mass. Regular exercise, especially weight-bearing activities, can help slow down these changes and keep us strong and mobile.

Heart Health

The heart works harder as we age. Blood vessels can become less flexible, increasing the risk of high blood pressure and heart disease. A healthy diet, regular exercise, and managing stress are crucial for maintaining heart health.

Vision Changes

It's no secret that as people age, their eyesight tends to alter. It gets difficult to read menus at dimly lit restaurants, and those reading glasses your older loved ones keep become their best friends. Age-related macular degeneration, cataracts, and a diminished capacity to focus on close objects (presbyopia) can all cause this alteration in vision. Having regular eye exams and, if necessary, wearing corrective lenses can help preserve healthy eyesight.

Hearing Loss

As one age, the world may appear a little quieter. Talk turns into a "What did they say?" game. It's not unusual, though, and getting regular screenings for hearing loss and, if required, wearing aids can help in living a better life.

Metabolism and Weight

It appears impossible to gaze upon a piece of cake without gaining weight, isn't that, right? Well, as people age, their metabolisms tend to slow down, which can facilitate weight gain. Maintaining a balanced diet and being physically active are important for controlling weight and general health.

Immune System

As people age, their immune systems may become less effective, leaving them more vulnerable to illnesses. Maintaining a healthy lifestyle and receiving regular immunizations are two ways to help the immune system.

Skin Changes

With age, changes to the skin occur, such as a slight loss of elasticity, dryness, and the appearance of age spots. Using moisturizers, drinking plenty of water, and shielding the skin from the sun can all help to keep skin healthy.

Oral Health

A person's oral health may require a little extra care as they become older. Problems like gum disease and tooth loss are not unusual. One can maintain a bright smile by scheduling routine dental exams, maintaining proper oral hygiene, and eating a well-balanced diet.

The Psychological Aspect of Aging

It's amazing how some people in their 80s can still clearly remember their twenties, while others could briefly forget the name of their grandchild. The answer, though, is inside our brains! As we become older, our brain goes through changes that have a significant impact on how our minds function.

As we age, cognitive decline is a natural part of the process, but it doesn't happen to everyone in the same way. It varies from person to person in terms of how much and how quickly it occurs. It's similar to how certain 60-year-olds may find it harder to remember things than certain vivacious 70-year-olds. And it gets even more intriguing: someone may have a photographic memory, yet they may struggle when it comes to making decisions.

This cognitive rollercoaster is like a large puzzle, with many factors contributing to its formation, including our biology, thoughts and emotions, general health, surroundings, and lifestyle choices. In light of this, let's examine a few of the symptoms:

- Slower Thinking: Problem-solving and thorough thought processes can occasionally become a little bit slower.

- Getting Lost Easier: It can get harder to maintain spatial orientation, such as knowing where you are.

- Perceptual Speed Bumps: You may have noticed that your perceptual speed - the capacity to process information quickly - isn't as swift as it once was.

- Math May Get Difficult: It may take a little more effort to crunch numbers.

- Memorable Moments: It could get harder to remember things like names or where the keys are.

- Language Retains Strength: It may surprise you to learn that verbal skills generally remain constant or even get better with age for some people.

These functions could change over time.[2] It's fascinating

---

[2] *The Biology of Aging.* sphweb. (n.d.).
https://sphweb.bumc.bu.edu/otlt/mph-modules/ph/aging/mobile_pages/aging5.html#:~:text=In%20general%2

to note that linguistic talents seem to hold up or even improve, while certain areas, like spatial orientation, may suffer. Thus, the ways in which our thoughts change throughout time are very diverse.

Cultural Lens on Aging

Culture isn't just about what you eat, what you wear, or how you celebrate. It's much more than that. Culture shapes who you are and has a big impact on how you see aging and how you care for older people.

Elders are revered in a lot of societies. For example, in Asian cultures, caring for elderly parents is a duty. On the other hand, some cultures focus more on youth and beauty, which can influence how older people are viewed and treated.

Different cultures have different ways of marking important life stages, especially aging. There are special ceremonies, traditions, and even rules for how to care for someone who is dying. Some families prefer to look after sick loved ones at home, while others choose to use hospitals or special care homes.

What people believe about health and how to stay well also affects how older people are cared for. Some cultures use old-fashioned healing methods, while others trust modern medicine.

How old people are expected to live their lives changes from place to place. In some places, older people keep working, while in others, they retire. These ideas affect how older people

---

C%20however%2C%20the%20symptoms,Declines%20in%20perceptu
al%20speed

feel about themselves and their money. It's important to remember that people from different cultures are mixing more. This means that old ways of thinking about aging are changing, and new ideas are being formed.

There's something very interesting about learning the different cultural backgrounds of our aging loved ones. It's an essential component of giving the greatest care possible, not just a nice touch. Consider it this way: by taking the time to learn about the customs, traditions, and cultural nuances of the elderly people we are taking care of, we can make sure that they receive care that genuinely suits their needs and preferences, in addition to treating them with respect.

In our world today, it's really important to learn about different people. It helps us give everyone the best care possible as they get older. So, if you're taking care of someone, try to learn about their culture. It's a kind thing to do.

The Growing Health Challenges

Our healthcare system needs to prepare for specific health concerns that are coming up as a result of the aging population. Among them are:

- Cancer: As the population ages, the number of instances of cancer is predicted to soar, reaching 27 million by 2030.[3]

- Dementia: It is also expected that the prevalence of dementia, especially Alzheimer's disease, will increase dramatically. By 2050, 115 million people are expected

---

[3] Suzman, R., & Beard, J. (2015). *Global health and aging:* preface. National Institute on Aging website.

to have dementia, with a large proportion of those affected living in less developed nations.

- Rise in Falls: Falls are a major source of injuries for senior citizens and are posing an increasing healthcare concern. This is becoming more and more of a concern as Baby Boomers live longer, are more active, and occasionally take drugs that raise their risk of falling. According to a survey published by the American Hospital Association (AHA), every year, more than one-third of seniors 65 years of age or older fall, and many of them have moderate to serious injuries such as hip fractures. By 2050, hip fracture rates are predicted to double.

- Obesity: An increasing proportion of people are overweight, which increases their risk of developing a number of illnesses.

- Diabetes: Another chronic illness that is increasing is diabetes. The American Heart Association (AHA) projects that by 2030, there will be 46 million Americans living with diabetes, a large share of whom are Baby Boomers.

To guarantee that our healthcare system can sufficiently serve an aging population, these health issues necessitate rigorous planning and initiatives. We need to be smart about how we take care of older people. One of the best ways is to stop problems before they start. This is called preventative care.

Imagine being able to do the things you love without getting sick all the time. That's what preventative care can do. It helps your elderly loved ones stay independent and enjoy their life.

Aging, to put it briefly, is a time of complexity and opportunity. It's about appreciating the special life experiences and embracing change. Therefore, as you proceed on this journey - whether you're taking care of your elderly parents or yourself as a professional caregiver - do it with empathy, understanding, and a dedication to upholding the dignity of those who've walked the road ahead of us.

Chapter 2: What Do Your Elderly Loved Ones or Patients Need and Want?

Growing older is a natural part of life. Our parents start to depend on us to help them through this new phase of aging, just as we have relied on them for love, support, and advice throughout our lives. The level of dependency could vary, but it's there. It's a dramatic change when our parents begin to rely on us in the same way that we once did. But why is it so important to take into account our parents' views and needs as they become older?

Well, understanding their aspirations and needs at a deeper level will allow you to build a new, more meaningful relationship with them and also help them in going through this aging journey a little easily. Your parents' needs, wants, and viewpoints change as they become older. Among many other issues, they might deal with limitations in their mobility, health issues, or a desire for greater independence. One part of this journey is realizing that people who have supported you through thick and thin, held your hand during times of anxiety, and applauded your victories are now asking for your help on their own path. This includes taking into consideration their hopes, their concerns, and their aspirations.

I have heard that your character is shown by how you treat those who can't do anything for you. Our parents, who gave us support and love, deserve our care and respect as they grow older. This is our chance to show our gratitude toward them. The journey ahead might have some bumps and uncertainties.

But by understanding and valuing your parents' views and wants as they age, you can create a loving and supportive environment for them to continue growing older with a bit of ease.

Communicate With Them

Having a conversation with your parents is just one part of this journey that is very important. As they age, they might need a bit more tender loving care, even if they don't always admit it. Discussing their future health and lifestyle can be challenging for everyone involved.

Conversations about caregiving or managing finances can be especially tough for the older generation. They often see it as a loss of their freedom and independence, which can be hard for them to accept. They might brush off your well-intentioned suggestions for all sorts of reasons – like not wanting to give up their say in decisions or letting others step in to help with their daily routines.

This is where having those tough conversations with aging loved ones becomes really important. Let's dive into this a bit more and explore some tips and strategies to help you during these discussions in an appropriate way.

1. Don't Wait for a Crisis

Talking about the future with your elderly loved ones can be tricky, especially if it's triggered by a sudden health scare. When your elderly are stressed, it's hard to look into what's ahead. So why not switch things up and be a bit more practical?

Instead of waiting for a crisis to come up, try to have these important conversations when your parents are relaxed and at ease. When they're not overwhelmed, it's easier to discuss the details and get their thoughts on how the family should handle things going forward.

2. <u>Try To Be Patient</u>

When you're preparing for sensitive conversations, it's really important to approach them with an open heart and a lot of patience. Setting strict expectations right from the start might not be the best approach. Your elderly loved ones might need some time to adjust to the changes that come with aging and might not be ready to talk about finances or caregiving just yet.

Start small and keep things simple. Give them gentle nudges and soft suggestions to show that you're there to support them. This helps them get used to the idea that you're available to help when needed. Don't be surprised if there's some resistance or if they try to avoid the topic at first. That's pretty normal, especially if they're not ready to accept help. However, if there are immediate health or financial risks, it's important to bring up the issue gently and persistently until you both can find a suitable solution.

3. <u>Choose the Perfect Setting</u>

Finding the right time and place for these dialogues is like setting the stage for a warm and open-hearted conversation. Pay attention to how your elderly respond during your regular chats to get a sense of their comfort zones. For discussions about things like caregiving choices and their legacy, choose a private, cozy, and calm setting.

Before starting the conversation, it's wise to have your goals and strategy clear, which would hopefully help in keeping the discussion focused and productive.

4. Pay Close Attention

During these critical discussions, it is important to keep in mind the value of actually listening to your elderly loved ones. Ask them questions like, *Are you hiding any suppressed feelings, such as anger or fear? Do you have regrets or unmet expectations that you would like to talk about? Are there still things you would like to accomplish in your later years?*

This is a great chance to help them come to terms with unsettled issues from the past and to identify resources and tools that can improve their quality of life now. Give priority to their sentiments by asking them about their feelings initially, then after they have had a chance to express themselves, put forward your honest suggestions.

5. Keep a Record

Discussions around end-of-life care and plans are continuing, and they can progress because of many factors like your elderly loved one's health, money, and mental state. During these conversations, it's a good idea to take notes so you can go over the information again when needed and modify your plan.

While guaranteeing your elderly's safety and access to the care they require is your top priority, it's also important to recognize and accept their concerns and objections as totally reasonable and legitimate. It might be unsettling to think about end-of-life care, so it's advised to approach the topic with compassion and reason and support them in making the best decisions possible.

Open Communication

Open communication has many benefits for normal human beings but it's especially valuable for seniors who struggle with loneliness and isolation. You can make a big difference in their mental and physical health and ultimately help in improving their quality of life when you listen well and engage them in conversation.

In addition, encouraging your senior loved one to stay active and maintain social connections can make a lot of difference. Research shows that seniors who spend more time with family and friends have better health and happiness, and they are less likely to suffer from chronic illnesses, anxiety, or depression.

Active Listening

We discussed earlier how paying attention and listening actively to your elderly loved ones is important. But it is equally imperative to mention here that active listening is not only important during these tough talks. Rather, it is a significant aspect of your entire caregiving journey.

Listening closely and attentively is a gold skill when caring for the elderly. Every now and then, what they're saying might not be the exact thing bothering them. For example, let's consider the following scenario. Your parent has been complaining about various physical aches and pains for weeks or even months. You have addressed some of these issues, perhaps resolved a problem or two, and assumed the complaining would stop. However, they continue to complain about aches and pains.

Here's where having keen listening skills comes into play. They may not be discussing their medical conditions; instead, they may be discussing something deeper that is difficult for them to express. Therefore, it's essential to delve a little farther, ask questions, and truly understand the root of their concerns.

Even if their words don't always convey the whole story, your ears might be able to decipher the real message.

When elderly people whine nonstop, it's usually not because they are in pain. Frequently, it's just a plain cry for company and someone who is willing to listen. Seniors often look for opportunities for connection, particularly if they feel alone or excluded from the daily commotion of life.

It's interesting just how often the elderly find themselves in this situation, needing only some companionship and understanding. They may not be asking you to fix their problems; all they need is for you to notice how they feel or to lend them a sympathetic ear when they talk about their sentiments.

Any changes to their communication style are something more to monitor. They may occasionally begin talking more or less than normal, which could indicate underlying anxiety or sadness. In other situations, they might speak in simpler terms, have memory problems, or have difficulty finding the correct words. They may even stop in the middle of a sentence and leave their thoughts unfinished.

These symptoms could be an early warning indication of Alzheimer's disease or even moderate cognitive impairments. It's highly important to recognize these changes and provide them with the understanding and support they require as soon as possible.

However, it's understandable that you're only human and can't always be by their side and the only person they confide in. If your elderly loved one has another caregiver, make sure to update them about the issue if they come by on a regular basis or from time to time. Tell them how much your loved one would gain from their listening abilities as well.

How Can You Become an Active Listener?

Your loved one's emotional health is equally as important as their physical health. When your senior loved one is talking, there's much more to active listening than just being silent. Sometimes, what they're worried about isn't obvious; it could be a fear of being left alone, worries about aging and health, or concerns about mental health.

Seniors often feel like they're not as important as they used to be or think they matter less to those around them. This is where active listening comes in. As they get older, their way of communicating might change a bit. But when you actively listen, it helps avoid misunderstandings and gives your elderly the confidence to share their feelings.

Active listening shows your seniors that they're valued and that you're dedicated to being the best caregiver possible. Through your actions, you're telling them, "You're important, and I'm here for you." Remember that being a good listener doesn't always mean having a back-and-forth conversation. Sometimes, just saying a word or two between the lines to show you're listening and understanding can make a big difference.

Managing Senior Emotions

A variety of typical worries and anxiety come along with aging. Identifying and understanding these worries is an important first step in providing emotional support to your elderly loved ones. As stated earlier, many elderly people are concerned about losing their independence and worry that they will want help with everyday chores that they used to complete on their own. Another common fear is that of becoming sicker since managing health issues may be overwhelming and extremely stressful.

Addressing Their Fears and Apprehensions

It's totally normal for your elderly loved ones to feel anxious about a few things, and understanding these concerns can help you support them better.

First up, loneliness and social isolation are big ones. Many seniors worry about losing touch with friends and family, which can make them feel really alone. Then there's the whole financial side of things. It's not uncommon for seniors to stress about having enough money to cover their future needs, especially when it comes to healthcare and daily living expenses. And, of course, the fear of cognitive decline or diseases like Alzheimer's is another major worry, as these conditions can seriously impact their daily lives.

So, what can we do to help? Well, actively listening is one thing that we discussed earlier that can help. Sometimes, just talking about these worries can make a big difference. And if things get too overwhelming, professional help from therapists or counselors who specialize in senior issues can be really beneficial.

Encouraging your parents to keep up their social connections is also important. Social activities and outings can really help in alleviating the fear of loneliness. For financial worries, helping in creating a solid financial plan can provide them with a sense of security and stability.

And let's not forget about promoting a healthy lifestyle! Regular physical activity, mental stimulation, and a balanced diet can go a long way in maintaining both physical and mental health.

Remember, it's important to acknowledge that these fears and feelings are completely normal. By reassuring your elderly and taking practical steps to address their concerns, you can make their aging process more manageable and make sure they feel loved and supported every step of the way.

Dealing with Control Issues

Caring for an aging or ill loved one is definitely a big challenge in itself, and it gets even tougher when they're being controlling. It's pretty common for elderly people to become a bit bossy about how and when things get done, which can really test the patience of family caregivers.

For example, you might observe that your elderly mom insists that you stay with her all the time but doesn't care about watching your favorite TV shows. Or your dad wants you to help with his personal care but flat-out refuses any professional help. Or maybe your spouse keeps complaining about the care and attention you give, no matter how hard you try.

It's important to understand that this controlling behavior often stems from a loss of independence. As they rely more on someone else, they might try to hold on to control in other ways. Recognizing this can really help in dealing with their demands and managing their behavior. By keeping this in mind, you can better handle the situation and respond to their needs in a way that makes both of you feel more at ease.

The Toll of Aging

People frequently feel that they're losing control as they age, particularly in terms of their independence. When your body isn't as strong as it once was and you have mobility problems or chronic pain, it might become difficult. Incontinence can make it difficult to even walk about at times, and it can be very embarrassing.

It can be exhausting to feel ill and not like yourself at any age. However, because there is frequently little that can be done to make things better, it can be very upsetting for elders. Depression may result from this knowledge, and the person receiving care from you may become resentful of those around them.

Ultimately, some elderly people begin controlling everything and everyone in their immediate surroundings as a somewhat maladaptive coping mechanism. And guess what? They may take it out on you, their caregiver, believing that you won't abandon them. Acknowledging that they are experiencing hardship and mourning can assist you in managing their incessant need to be in charge of everything.

Striking a Balance

It can be challenging to strike a balance between a senior's desire for control and their safety, particularly if that demand seems to be a coping mechanism for their irritation and anxiety. But to understand, try to place yourself in their position for a moment. Just picture someone who, even with the best of intentions, decided everything for you all of a sudden. Instead of actively participating in your own life, you would probably feel like a spectator.

It's critical to examine your own actions as a caregiver to determine whether you may be exerting more control than is required. Even when it's not necessary, caregivers occasionally step in because it's more effective. So, it could be wise to take a step back in certain situations.

Quite obviously, it can be annoying to wait for Mom to decide what to wear each morning or for Dad to select what to have for supper, but it's also important to give them autonomy over the tasks they can perform on their own. It's about striking a balance between their need for safety and their autonomy to make life decisions.

Are You and Your Loved One Teaming Up for Their Care?

Choosing senior care can be a very complicated process, and there are many aspects that play a role in it. Furthermore, limited life expectancy and age-related changes in mental and physical ability might complicate matters even further.

You and your elderly loved one need to talk openly and often about short- and long-term healthcare goals in order to make the best decisions. This entails collaborating closely with doctors and other healthcare providers as well as the full care team. You may confidently and thoroughly evaluate all of the care options by doing this.

Shared Decision-making

Using a hypothetical scenario, let's examine what collaborative decision-making might look like. Imagine that your aging mother is suffering from a severe case of Parkinson's disease (PD), which has left her unable to walk, eat, or dress herself. She recently saw her doctor and was told that she had been diagnosed with stage IV colon cancer. In addition to treatment, the doctor advises surgery to remove the tumor from her colon and any adjacent organs.

There are substantial dangers associated with both surgery and chemotherapy, including the possibility of cognitive issues getting worse and, in extreme cases, even death. The doctors communicated that she has very little chance of surviving longer than six months, even with aggressive treatment. Parkinson's disease was rapidly lowering her quality of life, and undergoing cancer treatment would only make things worse on the physical and emotional levels. So, what seems like the wisest course of action?

This kind of situation is not uncommon among elders and the family caregivers who look after them. The best method considered for reaching difficult decisions regarding care is a process known as 'shared decision-making.' This process is a key component of patient-centered care, which entails prioritizing the elder's choices and values while determining the optimal course of treatment.

For the hypothetical scenario in point, the main question is: What is more important to your mother? Is it to make her last days as comfortable as possible, or is it to try to extend her life for a few more months?

As a family caregiver, your responsibility in shared decision-making depends on your loved one's capacity to actively engage in their own care and their openness to receiving assistance. When a senior's caregiver becomes very involved in their medical decisions, it's usually because the patient has physical or mental issues that make it difficult for them to make decisions on their own. In such circumstances, it becomes imperative to appoint a family caregiver as the senior's durable medical power of attorney (POA), which enables them to make choices on the senior's behalf.

Even while a senior has the capacity to make their own decisions, there are situations in which you can still have a significant influence in the process. Seniors frequently want their carers to be active in order to receive support and to be updated about their condition. You can play a crucial role as an advocate for your aging loved one by posing queries and speaking about your worries that might not have been brought up otherwise.

The next step in the scenario we have been taking into account would be to find out if your mother would like you to participate in the decision-making. Does she want to talk to you honestly and openly about the difficult topics surrounding her diagnosis? Does she have the legal capacity to decide how she will be treated? If not, do you possess the legal capacity to make choices on her behalf - for example, by being named as her durable medical power of attorney? As you work together to go through this challenging situation, these are some critical questions to address.

Collecting Information

You can actively participate in the shared decision-making process by being educated, which is an important part of it. Before visits, it can be very helpful to investigate your loved one's health, the treatments that are available, and the many types of care that are accessible. In addition to giving patients and doctors more control, it also shortens appointment times by removing the need for the doctor to describe every aspect of a given condition.

Pre-appointment research gives you, the caregiver, and the patient the opportunity to formulate specific queries and worries for the doctor to address. The internet has changed the game in recent years by making medical information more accessible and assisting patients and caregivers in becoming more informed. You can investigate your loved one's diagnosis and possible therapies with a few clicks. Online forums and support groups can also help you connect with people who have experienced similar medical problems and gain insightful knowledge from their own experiences.

But when it comes to conducting research online, there are a few things to remember. The internet is a mixed bag since anything may be posted there with barely any oversight. There is a wealth of information available, both good and bad. The source of such knowledge is what matters most. You may typically rely on information from reputable sources, such as the Alzheimer's Association, the Centers for Disease Control, official government websites, or reputable medical institutes, to be accurate and up-to-date.

So, for the case in point, what exact technical details regarding your mother's condition and treatment do you require? Acquiring this data will assist you in evaluating the benefits and drawbacks of alternatives such as surgery, chemotherapy, or alternative treatments.

Having Regular Conversations About Care Decisions

Actually, studies have revealed that not all patients like to have in-depth conversations about the specifics of possible treatments with their physicians. Some elderly people may only want to have faith in the medical knowledge of their doctor. Many elderly people develop relationships with their doctors in which the patient follows the doctor's advice, and the doctor takes the lead.

The truth is that a person's involvement in the decision-making process can also be influenced by their family relationships and cultural background. For instance, shared decision-making is frequently valued in Eastern cultures. Before a choice is made, family members are given the opportunity to voice their opinions. Thus, an aged person may occasionally defer to their family to assess the advantages and disadvantages and make the final decision.

It's true that not all healthcare decisions call for an extended dialogue on the values and aims of the patient. But a lot of the medical problems that older adults deal with are complicated enough to require an in-person discussion with important caregivers. Surprisingly, though, the medical community doesn't use shared decision-making nearly as frequently as it ought to.

A patient's values and treatment objectives are rarely discussed during a doctor's appointment, which is typically only 15 to 20 minutes long. But in certain situations, if you and your loved one want to talk about a topic in greater detail, you should definitely speak up. In fact, most physicians find it simpler to interact when they are aware that the patient and caregiver are interested in learning more.

It is important to remember that, unless there is an urgent medical emergency, shared decision-making is not limited to one big medical choice. As a senior's disease progresses, their objectives may also change. Because of this, it's important to have continuing discussions to make sure that their care plan continues to reflect their changing preferences and goals. Over time, if you maintain an open line of communication, the entire care team will have a deeper grasp of your senior's priorities and preferred method of care.

End-of-Life Care Decisions

Many shared decision-making conversations with older loved ones center on end-of-life care. This often means deciding on the best way to handle a serious illness: whether to pursue aggressive treatment, opt for palliative care, or choose hospice care.

Being involved in these decisions is both an honor and a significant responsibility. It can be hard to honor someone's wishes while also dealing with your own feelings about losing them. Open and honest conversations about end-of-life preferences are vital before a medical crisis arises. Advanced care planning, including documents like a power of attorney for healthcare, might help. However, it's important to remember that these documents might not always reflect a person's true wishes. Therefore, ongoing conversations are very important.

Talking about end-of-life care can be difficult, but it's never too early to start considering and talking about things, particularly if a loved one is just beginning to show signs of dementia. It's important to honor the autonomy of your senior loved ones. It involves giving them freedom of choice and doing everything in your power to respect their desires, all the while ensuring their safety and comfort. It's about letting them make their own decisions about their lives but also being there to support and guide them. Finding this balance shows you care and helps them keep their dignity and autonomy.

Chapter 3: The Physical Needs Are Important!

Just like you would check your loved one's blood pressure or heart rate, it's important to think about their general health as well. When you care for elderly family members, you might want to think about what being healthy means for them and if they're meeting those goals. Here are some simple questions to help you see how they're doing:

Do they like being active and exercising?

Do they have friends or family to do activities with?

Are they making time to stay active?

Are they looking after their physical health?

Are they eating healthy, nutritious foods?

Are they moving around enough?

How does their health stack up against others their age?

If you answered "no" to any of these, it might mean there's room for improvement in their physical health.

Mobility and Balance

Mobility is one of the things that makes life a bit easier. It's the freedom to move around, play, and explore. But as we get older, it can sometimes become harder to do the things we love. You might notice changes in your loved one's posture, walking, or energy levels. They might feel tired or weak or have trouble getting in and out of chairs. These changes are normal parts of aging. Muscles can get weaker, bones can become thinner, and joints can stiffen.

As caregivers, understanding these changes is important. It can help us support our loved ones in staying active and safe. By encouraging regular exercise, discussing safety tips, and helping with mobility aids when needed, we can make a big difference in their quality of life.

Research shows that limited mobility can greatly increase the risk of becoming dependent on others for daily activities. This is because mobility is important for tasks like attending appointments, participating in social activities, etc. The more your elderly loved ones become dependent, the more there would be chances for a need for long-term care, which can have a deep effect on their health.

Tools for Improving Mobility

So, the goal is to simply help our elderly loved ones stay independent and active. To do that, we need to keep an eye on their mobility and balance. Here are some simple ways to check on these things:

- *Watch and Observe:* Watch how your senior moves during daily activities like walking, getting up from a chair, sitting down, and turning. Look for signs of instability or any changes in how they usually move.

- *Physical Examination:* Healthcare providers can check muscle strength, joint flexibility, and balance through a full physical exam. They'll look for things like weak muscles, stiff joints, and how well the person can keep their balance in different positions.

- *Timed Up and Go (TUG) Test:* This is a quick and easy way to evaluate mobility. It works by having your loved one sit in a chair they use every day. When you say "go," they get up, walk about 10 feet, turn around, and come back to sit down. You time how long it takes them to do this.

If they take longer than 12 seconds or seem unsteady, it might mean they need some help with their mobility and balance.

- *Berg Balance Scale:* This test goes a bit further than the TUG test by providing a more detailed look at a person's balance and mobility. It includes 14 different tasks, like standing on one foot or reaching for something while sitting. Each task is scored based on how well your loved one can perform it. If they do the task easily, they get a higher score. If they struggle or need help, they receive a lower score, which means more balance issues.

- *Gait Assessment:* This test looks into an elderly's gait or how they walk. Here's what you can look out for:

  o Speed: Notice how fast or slow they walk. Are they moving at a comfortable pace, or do they seem unusually fast or slow?

  o Stride Length: Watch the length of their steps. Are their steps stable and even, or are they irregular?

  o Balance: Pay attention to their balance as they walk. Are they wobbly, stumbling, or veering to one side?

  o Coordination: See if they're swinging their arms in sync with their steps. Lack of coordination can indicate mobility issues.

  o Foot Clearance: Check how high they lift their feet with each step. If they're dragging or shuffling their feet, it could signal mobility difficulties.

o Symmetry: Look to see if their steps are even and symmetrical or if they have an uneven gait.

If you notice anything concerning, it's a good idea to talk to your loved one's doctor to see if any exercises or interventions are needed.

- *Functional Reach Test:* This test is pretty simple and doesn't need any special equipment. Here's how you do it:

    o Have your loved one stand next to a wall, about shoulder-width away.

    o Ask them to stretch their arm out in front of them at shoulder height, parallel to the floor.

    o Without moving their feet, they reach as far forward as they can without losing their balance or lifting their heels.

    o You measure the distance from where they started to where they reached.

This test is all about seeing how well they can keep their balance while reaching. The farther they can reach, the better their balance. If they have trouble reaching far or seem wobbly, it might mean they could use some extra help with balance and mobility.

- *Fall Risk Assessment:* These valuations look at different factors that could grow the risk of falling, like the medications they're on, any medical history they have, and any vision or hearing problems. A higher score here might mean a greater risk of falls.

- *Home Safety Assessment:* This assessment is all about making sure your elderly loved one's home is a safe place. It starts with checking the lighting, flooring, stairs, etc. Bathrooms can be a tricky spot, and so can the kitchen. Clearing walkways of clutter and securing any loose cords are also important ways to help prevent them from falling.

- *Cognitive Assessment:* Sometimes, problems with thinking or memory can affect how well someone moves or balances. One common tool for this is the Mini-Mental State Examination (MMSE), which is a quick test that checks things like memory, simple math, and awareness of the surroundings. Other tests might be used to look at specific cognitive functions. These assessments are important because they can help in figuring out if thinking or memory problems are contributing to mobility issues.

- *Collaboration with Specialists:* Getting help from specialists like physical therapists, occupational therapists, and orthopedic doctors can provide you with a deeper understanding of the issues and help create a personalized treatment plan for your elderly. For instance, physical therapists can develop exercise programs custom-made to look after particular challenges of your elderly loved one's mobility and balance.

- *Balance and Strength Training:* Exercise programs should be customized to fit your loved one's needs and abilities. These might include balance exercises, like standing on one leg, and strength training, such as using resistance bands or weights.

- *Medication Review:* Some medications can cause dizziness or affect balance. Your elderly's doctor can review their medications to spot any possible issues and suggest alternatives with fewer side effects.

Management of Chronic Illness

As people get older, they're more likely to face health problems that aren't as common in younger people. There are conditions like high blood pressure, heart disease, urinary incontinence, dementia, and multiple sclerosis that usually show up more often in older people. Sometimes, high blood pressure runs in families and can affect different generations.

Many older people have one or more chronic health conditions. In fact, most people over 65 have at least one, and many have more than one. Chances are, you might know a parent or grandparent dealing with one of these conditions. While some changes, like eyesight problems or hearing loss, are normal as we age, it's important to remember that not all health issues are just part of getting older. Some things might be caused by other factors that need to be addressed.

Let's take a closer look at some of the health issues older people often face.

- *Arthritis:* Arthritis is one of the most common issues, especially for those 65 and older. It can cause pain and make it harder to move, which can make everyday activities more difficult.

- *Heart Disease:* Heart disease can show up in many ways, including problems with cholesterol, blood pressure, and other heart-related issues. It's a common problem for people aged 60 and up.

- *Diabetes:* This is a disease that affects how the body uses blood sugar. It can cause high blood sugar levels and can be difficult to manage. There are three main types of diabetes, including Type 1 Diabetes, which usually starts in childhood or adolescence and needs insulin treatment; Type 2 Diabetes, which is the most common type and is usually related to lifestyle and can be managed with medication, diet, and exercise and; Gestational Diabetes, which happens during pregnancy and needs careful monitoring.

- *Chronic Kidney Disease (CKD):* This is a common problem in seniors. It's when the kidneys slowly stop working well. CKD can be caused by high blood pressure, diabetes, or age-related changes. The risk of CKD increases as people get older, often progresses slowly, and may not be noticed until it's advanced.

- *Chronic Obstructive Pulmonary Disease (COPD):* This is a lung disease that can cause breathing problems. It's common in older people and is often a result of long-term exposure to irritants like cigarette smoke. COPD can affect the daily activities and mobility of the elderly.

- *Osteoporosis:* This is a disease that weakens bones and makes them more likely to break. It's common in older people, especially postmenopausal women. Osteoporosis often doesn't have symptoms until a fracture happens. Elderly people with osteoporosis have a higher risk of fractures, which can affect their mobility.

- *Dementia and Alzheimer's Disease:* These are conditions that can affect seniors. Alzheimer's disease is a type of dementia that affects 11% of older people. It causes memory loss and problems with thinking and problem-solving. Please remember that dementia is not a normal part of aging.

Age, family history, and genetics can make the risk of many chronic illnesses higher. However, lifestyle changes can help in delaying or preventing these conditions.

Tracking and Handling Chronic Illness

Chronic health conditions usually stick around for life. These conditions can be managed, but they need regular check-ins and monitoring. Regular checkups with doctors, routine tests, and managing medications are all parts of this process. If you keep a close eye on things, chances are that you will be able to catch any changes in your elderly's health early on. Early detection can prevent complications and make symptoms less severe. If these conditions aren't observed, they can lead to complications like nerve damage or vision problems with diabetes.

While observation and everything else is important, please remember that medical care is not the only thing to look into. Lifestyle choices like eating a balanced diet and getting regular exercise are also important for managing chronic illnesses. You can consider these habits as the rudders that keep a ship moving in the right direction. Your job is to make sure these lifestyle changes are working well and are sustainable for your elderly loved one.

Medication Matters

You already know that meds are important for your elderly's health. But when they're not feeling well or have many pills to take, it can be hard to keep track. If they forget to take meds, it can make things worse. Their quality of life might not improve, and sometimes, it can even get worse. So, it's important to make sure they take their meds on time and follow their doctor's instructions, especially when you can't be there to help. Your care can make a big difference in their lives.

Medication management is a service that helps people like your elderly stay on top of their medications. The goal is to make sure they take their meds as prescribed every time and avoid any problems from taking them wrong. You'll every so often find this service in assisted living facilities and senior living communities. You might also hear terms like 'medication adherence' and 'medication compliance.'

For some people, a simple reminder device might work. But for others, a more complete system of reminders and help is needed. In many assisted living settings, residents get medication management services from trained teams. They make sure all prescriptions are filled on time and all meds are taken correctly each day.

Medication Compliance Strategies

It can be hard to keep track of all the meds your elderly loved one needs. However, you can help them stick to their medication routine, which can make a big difference in their health and quality of life. Here are some ways to help them with medication management:

- *Simplify Their Meds:* Talk to their doctor about making their medications as simple as possible. Fewer meds and taking them less often can make it easier to remember.

- *Use Pill Organizers:* Get your loved ones a pill organizer with compartments for each day of the week or at different times of the day. This can help them remember when to take their medications and avoid any mix-ups.

- *Review Meds Regularly:* Have regular checkups with their doctor to make sure their meds are still right for them and to check for any side effects.

- *Get Meds at Once:* Try to get all their medications refilled at the same time. This makes it less likely they'll forget to take something.

- *Label Meds Clearly:* Make sure the labels on their medicines are easy to read. For people with vision problems, use large-print labels.

- *Use Technology:* Use smartphone apps or specialized medication management devices that can set up reminders and even dispense medications at the right time.

- *Educate Them:* Give your parents or elderly loved one information about their meds, including side effects and why they need to take them.

- *Store Meds Safely:* Keep meds away from kids and pets, and in a cool, dry place.

- *Watch for Side Effects:* Tell their doctor about any unusual side effects or symptoms.

- *Get Specialized Packaging:* Some pharmacies offer special packaging services, like blister packs, that organize medications by dose and time.

Nutritional Needs of the Elderly

Good nutrition is really important for everyone, especially as we get older. Eating healthy can help manage illnesses and other health problems. Knowing what a healthy diet is and paying attention to what your elderly eat can make a big difference in their health. A balanced diet gives energy, helps control weight, and can even prevent diseases like heart disease, high blood pressure, type 2 diabetes, osteoporosis, and certain cancers.

As your elderly get older, their bodies and lifestyles change. This means they might need different foods than when they were younger. They might need less energy but more protein. What works for younger people might not be right for older people.

Our bodies need the right nutrients to work best. These nutrients come from the food we eat. The main nutrients we need are proteins, carbohydrates, and fats, which are like the building blocks that our bodies use to do different things. It is important to make sure your parents get the right balance of these nutrients and stay hydrated.

A well-proportioned diet is usually about eating a variety of natural, wholesome foods, which include fruits, vegetables, whole grains, dairy, and protein sources. Choose lean meat and poultry and low-fat dairy products.

It's also important to avoid overly processed foods and high-sodium options. Watch their fat and cholesterol intake to make sure their diet is healthy. Remember, micronutrients like vitamins and minerals are also important, even in small amounts. Let's have a look at some key dietary considerations to help your elderly stay well:

- *Calcium and Vitamin D:* These are important for bone health. Encourage your elderly to eat three servings of low-fat or fat-free dairy products daily. They can also get calcium from dark green leafy vegetables, fortified cereals, fruit juices, canned fish, and fortified plant-based beverages. Vitamin D is found in fatty fish, eggs, and fortified foods and drinks.

41

- *Vitamin B12:* With age, it can be harder to absorb Vitamin B12. Suggest them options like seafood, lean meats, fish, and fortified cereals to help them get enough.

- *Dietary Fiber:* Fiber can help in reducing the risk of diabetes and heart disease. Encourage your senior to eat foods like whole-grain bread, cereals, lentils, beans, peas, whole vegetables, and fruits.

- *Potassium:* Potassium can help in lowering blood pressure. You can include foods like beans, vegetables, fruits, and low-fat dairy products in the diet of your elderly.

- *Polyunsaturated and Monounsaturated Fats:* These healthy fats can be found in vegetable oils, seeds, nuts, avocados, and fish. They're good for overall health.

Another important thing to consider here is the hydration of your senior. We all know how important water intake is for ourselves. It is so important for young people, then you can imagine the benefits for the older generations.

The easiest way to keep hydrated is by drinking water. Experts suggest about six to eight glasses a day for adults. But it doesn't necessarily have to be just plain water. Milk, juice, and tea count, too, and can help keep them hydrated.

The trick is making sure they keep drinking throughout the day. Dehydration can really complicate existing health issues or even lead to new ones, and we definitely want to steer clear of that.

How to Take Care of Their Dietary Challenges?

You may have noticed your senior making trouble while eating. It can range from them eating too little, being picky, or just not eating at all. So, let's briefly look into how you can tackle these challenges.

- *Chewing Issues:* If chewing is tough for them, it might be time for a dental checkup. Dental problems can sometimes be the culprit.

- *Help with Swallowing:* Ask your senior to drink plenty of liquids with their meals. If that doesn't help, talk to their doctor. There might be other health issues or medications causing problems.

- *Get Creative with Food:* If their senses of smell and taste are changing, make their food look and feel different. You can try to add colors and different textures to make it appealing to them.

- *Nutrient Intake:* If they're not eating enough, try giving them healthy snacks throughout the day, which can help them get more nutrients and calories in small portions.

- *Fight Loneliness:* It's very possible that your parents might be feeling lonely and that's one of the reasons they don't eat much. You might have noticed it yourself that when you eat with the people you love or within a comfortable group setting, you end up eating more. The same might be the case with your senior. So, you can consider having potluck meals with friends or cooking together and eating together. You can also check out nearby senior centers or community centers that offer meals.

- *Problem due to an illness:* If your elderly loved one is having trouble cooking or eating due to illness or health issues, don't hesitate to talk to their doctor. They might suggest an occupational therapist who can help them find ways to make meal prep and eating easier.

Pain Management

It can be hard to know if an older person is in pain since everyone expresses their pain in different manners. Some choose to say it in words, and some do not, and when they do not, it can be hard to identify. But with a little attention and care, you can really make a difference.

The Problems with Identifying Pain

Verbal Communication:

Some seniors do not express their pain verbally. In that case, you would need to pay close attention to their non-verbal cues. Look for small signs like changes in their facial expressions, body language, or behavior. For example, if they're wincing, frowning, or seeming more withdrawn than usual, it might be a sign that something is bothering them.

Be empathetic and let them know you're there for them. Ask them to share their feelings without pressuring them to talk if they're not ready. Sometimes, just knowing that you're attentive and caring can provide a lot of comfort to them.

Instead of asking yes or no questions, try open-ended ones that invite them to share more, like, "How have you been feeling lately? Can you tell me more about it?" This style gives them the space to open up at their own pace.

Multiple Health Conditions:

Many elderly people deal with several health issues at once, which can make it tough to figure out exactly where the pain is coming from. Don't hesitate to reach out to their doctor for help. Also, keeping a record of their symptoms, medications, and any changes you notice can be very useful. This information will help doctors make a more accurate assessment. Keep the lines of communication open with your parents' healthcare team and share any concerns, observations, and questions you have.

Fear of Burdening Others:

Many older adults don't want to complain because they fear being a burden to their loved ones. Let your parents know you truly care about them. Show your concern for their comfort and reassure them that you're there to support them.

In these situations, it might be helpful to ask direct questions. Seniors might not speak up because they don't want to worry anyone. You can ask specific questions about their comfort or pain, like, "Is there anything bothering you today?" or "Are you in any pain?"

When your parents do open up, listen carefully and without judgment. Their willingness to share should be met with empathy and understanding. Whenever possible, you can offer options for care or activities that let them make decisions about their own comfort.

Side Effects of Medicines

Sometimes, medicines can cause pain or other problems, which is why you need to learn about the medicines your parents take. Ask their doctor about side effects and if there are other medicines they can try. Usually, a small adjustment in medication can make a huge difference in your senior's life and comfort.

Cognitive Challenges:

If your parents have dementia, then I can understand how difficult it would be to deal with them. Cognitive decline can make it hard for your loved ones to express their pain or discomfort. Be patient and remember that their ability to communicate might be limited.

Keep a close eye on any changes in their behavior, as these can usually signal pain. They might show their discomfort through actions and body language rather than words. If they seem restless, agitated, or withdrawn, it could be a sign of distress.

Effective Pain Management Strategies

How we feel emotionally can have a big influence on how we go through pain and feel it. That's why it's so important to understand what might be the reason behind your elderly loved one's pain and to find some practical ways to help them manage it.

Pain Medications

Pain medications come in many forms, and they work in different ways to help in relieving discomfort. Here's a simple way to understand them, especially if you're caring for elderly parents.

NSAIDs (Nonsteroidal Anti-Inflammatory Drugs) like aspirin are commonly used to manage pain. They reduce inflammation and fever. On the other hand, opioid medications work differently from NSAIDs. They change the way pain messages are sent to the brain and provide powerful pain relief. Nevertheless, they also have a budding for addiction, so it's important to use them only under the guidance of a doctor to make sure they are taken as prescribed.

Heat or Cold Therapy

Sometimes, the simplest things can make a big difference. When it comes to managing pain, heat and cold therapy can be very helpful.[4] If your elderly have sprained their ankle or strained a muscle, reach for the ice pack. Cold therapy lowers the temperature of the skin and muscles, which helps slow blood flow and metabolic activity. This cooling effect reduces inflammation and swelling, which can alleviate pain.

For chronic pain like arthritis or persistent muscle aches, heat can be good. It helps to relax muscles and increase blood flow. Just be sure the heat isn't too hot, as it can cause burns, particularly in people who may have reduced sensitivity due to age. Use a moderate and comfortable level of warmth.

Deciding whether to use heat or cold depends on the type of pain you're dealing with. To put it simply, cold is great for new injuries, while heat is better for continuing aches and pains.

Physical Therapies

Physical therapies don't have to be complicated. As a matter of fact, everyday activities like walking, stretching, and gentle exercises can make a big difference in your elderly loved ones' lives.

---

[4] Lemiska, E. (2021). The benefits of heat and cold therapy for chronic pain. U.S. Pain Foundation. https://uspainfoundation.org/news/the-benefits-of-heat-and-cold-therapy-for-chronic-pain/

Walking is a simple but very beneficial way to reduce pain[5] as it helps improve blood circulation and can make joints and muscles feel less stiff. Plus, it's a great way to get some fresh air and boost your mood. Moreover, regular stretching can help prevent stiffness and improve flexibility. It's a gentle way to relax muscles and relieve tension. Along with this, building muscle strength can provide better support and stability. Start slowly and gradually increase the intensity to avoid overdoing it.

Massage Therapy

Massage therapy can be a wonderful addition to your elderly's pain management toolkit, especially if they deal with ongoing pain. Massage therapy is linked to fewer physical or emotional limitations, better emotional health, increased energy and reduced fatigue, greater social interactions, and better overall healthiness.[6] It's important to understand when and how to use it, keeping your elderly' needs in mind. The gentle kneading and manipulation of muscles can help ease uneasiness and improve blood flow to the affected areas.

However, there are a few things to consider when choosing massage for your elderly loved ones' pain. Please note that while massage can be great for soft tissues, it's not always the

---

[5] Vanti, C., Andreatta, S., Borghi, S., Guccione, A. A., Pillastrini, P., & Bertozzi, L. (2019). The effectiveness of walking versus exercise on pain and function in chronic low back pain: a systematic review and meta-analysis of randomized trials. *Disability and rehabilitation*, *41*(6), 622-632.

[6] Munk, N., Kruger, T., & Zanjani, F. (2011). Massage therapy usage and reported health in older adults experiencing persistent pain. *The Journal of Alternative and Complementary Medicine*, *17*(7), 609-616.

best choice when pain is centered in the joints.

Cognitive Behavioral Therapy (CBT)

CBT is a psychological technique that might help with handling and lessening your aging loved one's pain. It focuses on the connection between thoughts, emotions, and behaviors and how these can impact pain perception.

CBT teaches the patient to identify and confront negative thoughts that might be contributing to their pain. By replacing these thoughts with more positive and realistic ones, they can gain a greater sense of control over their pain experience.

CBT also looks at the connection between feelings and actions. Anxiety or frustration, for instance, can make people act in ways that could make their pain worse. Your senior can adopt new behaviors and coping mechanisms that support a proactive and optimistic approach to pain management by being aware of these linkages.

Transcutaneous Electrical Nerve Stimulation (TENS) Therapy

TENS therapy might sound a bit technical, but it's actually quite straightforward. It includes using low-voltage electrical currents that pass through the skin via electrodes placed on the body. This gentle electrical stimulation activates the body's natural pain relief system, sort of like flipping a switch to turn on your body's internal pain-fighting mode.

The interesting thing about TENS is that it can trick the body into feeling less pain by blocking pain signals or stimulating the release of endorphins, which are the body's natural painkillers. However, TENS therapy doesn't work for everyone and isn't effective for all types of pain. But for some elderly people who haven't found relief with other treatments, it might make a difference. If your elderly loved one is struggling with pain and is open to trying new therapies, TENS might be a worthwhile option to consider.

Preventive Health Measures

It's a bit scary to think that less than half of older adults in the US are getting the preventive care they need. But the good news is that these services can make a huge difference in their overall health and comfort.

Preventive care includes screenings for hidden health problems. More often than not, health problems can silently creep in without any obvious signs. This is where screening comes into play, which includes screenings for conditions like specific types of cancers, high blood pressure, or high blood sugar levels, which every so often don't show any obvious symptoms.

It's important to be conscious of health problems that might not always be obvious. Some issues cause noticeable symptoms but can still be easily missed during routine checkups. So, you need to pay close attention to your loved one's mental and emotional health as well. Make sure to ask about how they're feeling emotionally, whether they've experienced any falls recently, or if there are any signs of alcohol misuse. These are everyday concerns that usually go unnoticed but can greatly impact their health.

When I talk about preventative care, I notice that most people simply think about catching illnesses early. But, in reality, it also involves taking steps to reduce the risk of future health problems. This is where vaccines and medications can be considered as one of the important aspects of your elderly's health journey. Let's take a closer look at vaccinations and screenings.

Vaccinations and Screenings

Screenings

Let us talk about screenings first. Elderly people who are generally healthy but have a family history of certain diseases can really benefit from regular screenings. These tests can be very helpful, especially when it comes to catching serious conditions early. Some cancers, like those of the breast, cervix, colon, and prostate, can be life-threatening. But the good news is that screenings are available to detect them early. If your family has a history of these cancers, these screenings become even more important.

Breast Cancer Screening:

The risk of breast cancer increases with age. If you're caring for someone between the ages of 50 and 74, it's important to make sure they have a mammogram every two years. Depending on the risk factors, their doctor might recommend more frequent screenings.

It's always good to talk to the doctor about any specific concerns that could affect how frequently these screenings should be done.

Colorectal Cancer Screening:

Colorectal cancer is another condition where early detection is important. Starting at age 50, adults should undergo regular colorectal cancer screenings, which can include fecal immunochemical tests, flexible sigmoidoscopy, or colonoscopy. Each of these methods has its own set of risks and benefits, so it's important to discuss with the doctor which one is best suited for your loved one.

Cholesterol Screening:

To reduce the risk of heart disease and stroke, men over 35 and women over 45 should have regular cholesterol checks. This is a simple blood test that can give a clear picture of heart health and help to avoid serious issues down the line.

Diabetes Screening:

You must have heard every third person being diagnosed with diabetes these days. Yes, that's how common it has become. If your senior is overweight, their doctor might suggest testing for diabetes, even if they aren't showing any obvious symptoms. Diabetes can be sneaky and may not always present clear signs, so early detection is important. Even if your loved ones feel fine, getting screened for diabetes, especially if they carry extra weight, is a smart move.

High Blood Pressure Screening:

Regular blood pressure checks are important for your loved ones, ideally at least once a year. With age, the risk of high blood pressure increases, which makes these routine checks important.

Osteoporosis Screening

As we get older, it's really important to take care of our bones. If we don't, we might get osteoporosis, which makes our bones weak and can lead to broken bones. A bone density test, which is called a 'bone mass' test, can help you find out if your elderly's bones are strong enough. If they catch osteoporosis early, you can do things to slow it down and prevent breaks.

Smoking History

If your elderly loved one is a person who used to smoke or currently smokes, it's a good idea to get checked for certain things. Smoking can make a person more likely to get problems like an abdominal aortic aneurysm or lung cancer. Regular screenings can find these issues early when they're easier to fix.

Vaccines

Our immune systems don't usually remain as strong with age, and they might take longer to recover from illnesses. That's why vaccines and booster shots are so helpful. Following are a few important vaccines to consider.

Tdap Vaccines: You should consider getting your elderly loved one Tdap vaccines, which protect against tetanus, diphtheria, and whooping cough. These diseases can be quite serious, so staying up-to-date with these vaccines helps keep them at bay.

Influenza Vaccine: Elderly people, especially those over 65, are at higher risk for serious complications from the flu. A flu shot each year can lower the chances of getting the flu.

Pneumococcal Vaccines: Pneumonia can be a big concern for your elderly loved ones. There are two important vaccines for preventing it: the pneumococcal polysaccharide vaccine (PPSV) and the pneumococcal conjugate vaccine (PCV13). It's a good idea for everyone over 65 to get these shots to keep their lungs healthy.

COVID Vaccines: I'm sure we all know about COVID by now. It is still a serious issue, especially for those over 85. COVID-19 vaccines and boosters are important, so make sure you and your elderly get vaccinated against it.

Physical Activity and Exercise

I'm pretty sure I don't have to write long paragraphs explaining the importance of exercise. We all know its extensive benefits. Just how important it is for us, it's also equally or you can say even more important for our elderly loved ones.

Regular exercise can help manage health problems like diabetes, obesity, and heart disease in your elderly. It also helps prevent conditions like osteoporosis and obesity. It doesn't matter if your elderly go for a walk in the park or a gym session; the main point of concern is that they stay active. Preferably, people of all ages should include both aerobic exercises (like walking or swimming) and strength exercises (like lifting weights) in their routines.

Counsel Your Elderly

You can help make the lives of your elderly loved ones a little easier, if not completely healthy. For starters, if they're over 65, you can ask them kindly and lovingly to quit smoking. Smoking is closely linked to a higher risk of cancer and heart problems, both of which can be dangerous.

Diet is another biggie. Eating a lot of processed foods and unhealthy fats is like inviting heart issues to the party, especially conditions like coronary heart disease. And when you mix poor eating habits with a lack of exercise, it really ups the risk of health troubles for your senior loved ones.

But not everything is bad news. With the right support and a little counseling, you can help them make healthier choices. Counseling can be really helpful, especially when it comes to breaking long-standing habits. If you or your loved ones need a little nudge in the right direction, reaching out to a physician for advice on quitting tobacco, improving nutrition, or getting more active can make a huge difference. Doctors have the know-how to create strategies that lead to lasting, positive changes.

And let's not forget about preventive care. Not only is it about feeling better but also about saving on healthcare costs in the long run. Being proactive about health - whether it's yours or your loved ones' - means you're not just taking care of today but also trying to stay healthy tomorrow.

Part II:
Love, Loss, and Dementia

Chapter 4: Demystifying Dementia

Cognitive health plays a major role in our health, especially as we age. When we talk about cognitive needs, we're really looking at how the brain functions day to day, basically things like memory, problem-solving, and attention. For many of us, these skills help us go through life smoothly. But when cognitive health dwindles over time, it can affect everything from a person's independence to their emotional health. People taking care of the elderly who are losing their cognitive health slowly over time probably understand this very clearly.

Understanding the shifts is important. For instance, Dementia can change how someone experiences the world around them, which can make simple tasks difficult to carry out and sometimes very overwhelming. When your elderly's brain is working well, they can enjoy activities, make decisions, and stay connected with the people around them. But when cognitive health declines, even the simplest things can become tough.

Staying mentally sharp helps seniors keep their independence. They can remember appointments or chat with their friends without needing your help. When cognitive health fades, it can lead to frustration or sadness as everyday tasks become more difficult, which can affect not only how they see themselves but also their relationships and their loved ones.

The Silent Progression

While caring for your elderly loved ones, you might start noticing small changes in their thinking and memory. These changes can happen slowly, and at first, they might seem like normal aging. It's common for people to have some trouble remembering things or learning new information as they get older. But, for some people, these signs might point to something more, like Alzheimer's disease.

For example, they may start to forget names or events more often, take longer to learn new things or get distracted easily. You might also see them needing more time to understand new information or finding it hard to do more than one thing at a time. While these changes can feel like normal aging to you, it's important to keep an eye on them.

I want to emphasize here that we need to pay attention to these shifts as caregivers to our elderly loved ones. You can notice things like them losing track of time, misplacing items, or struggling to follow a conversation. These can be early signs that something more serious is going on. If you notice things like these, it might be a good idea to talk to a doctor and get the right support. More importantly, remember that this process might require a lot of patience from your end since these changes can be confusing or frustrating for your loved one.

With time, our understanding of Alzheimer's disease has grown, and so researchers have discovered that the disease progresses through three main stages, known as the Alzheimer's Disease Continuum. These stages help us understand how the disease develops over time, from no visible signs to noticeable changes in thinking and memory. The three main phases are as follows:

Phase 1: Cognitively Normal (Preclinical Stage)

In the first phase, known as the cognitively normal or preclinical stage, people show no visible signs of memory problems or other cognitive decline. They continue to function normally in daily life, with no issues related to memory, language, or problem-solving. But even though there are no outward symptoms, recent research shows that changes in the brain can start years before Alzheimer's symptoms surface.[7]

In this phase, researchers are focused on finding biological markers, such as changes in brain structure or certain proteins, that could indicate a higher risk of developing Alzheimer's. The hope is to catch the disease before it progresses to give us the best chance to slow or stop its development.

Phase 2: Mild Cognitive Impairment (MCI)

The second stage of Alzheimer's disease is called mild cognitive impairment (MCI). This is when a person starts having more noticeable memory or thinking problems than what's normal for their age. They might have trouble remembering things, focusing, or making decisions. While MCI doesn't always lead to dementia, it can be an early sign.

Researchers are working hard to find ways to slow the disease during this phase, with the hope of delaying or even preventing dementia from developing. [8]

Phase 3: Dementia

Severe Dementia is the final and most severe phase of Alzheimer's disease. At this point, memory loss, confusion, and

---

[7] Alzheimer's Therapeutic Research Institute. (n.d.). *Understanding the Alzheimer's continuum*. USC.
https://atrinews.usc.edu/resources/understanding-the-alzheimers-continuum/
[8] See Footnote 7.

other thinking problems make daily tasks really difficult. People with dementia might struggle with things like getting dressed, preparing meals, or even recognizing the faces of the people they know – even yourself. Caring for someone with dementia can be very challenging, and they often need help from healthcare professionals to support both the person and their caregivers.

Right now, humans have found no cure for Alzheimer's or dementia, but ongoing research is working to find ways to ease symptoms and improve the quality of life for those affected.

Alzheimer's is a tough and complex disease that affects millions of people around the world. Understanding these three stages will help you recognize the early signs and manage the symptoms as best as you can. Early detection and support can make a big difference in improving the quality of life for you as well as your loved ones.

Normal Aging Vs. Dementia

As we get older, it's normal for some of our thinking abilities to slow down a bit. For example, around age 30, things like how fast we process information, how long or how much we stay focused, and remember details can start to change slowly. You might notice it becomes a little harder to multitask or find the right words. This happens because certain parts of the brain, like the hippocampus and the frontal and temporal lobes, shrink slightly with age.

But it's not all downhill! Some thinking skills, like vocabulary, reading, and reasoning, can actually stay the same or even get better as we age.

So, here comes the part where understanding the difference between normal aging and dementia comes in.

While it's natural to have small shifts in how quickly we think or focus, dementia is not part of normal aging. Dementia takes in more serious cognitive problems, like forgetting things quickly, trouble solving problems, or getting lost in places a person once knew, like their neighborhood. It can also affect how someone interacts socially or their physical coordination, like experiencing more falls or tremors.

It can sometimes be tricky to know when these changes are cause for concern, as everyone ages differently. What might seem like a big issue for one person could be normal for someone else, which actually makes it tough to figure out when to look for help.

Abnormal Aging

When we talk about abnormal aging, there are two key terms to know: Mild Cognitive Impairment (MCI) and dementia, as we discussed previously. MCI means that someone is starting to experience changes in their thinking, but these changes don't yet interfere with daily activities like cooking or driving. Dementia, however, means that cognitive decline has developed to a point where it affects their ability to handle everyday tasks.

So, it is important for you to know the difference between normal aging, MCI, and dementia so that it can help you better understand what's going on with your elderly loved ones and when it might be time to seek extra support.

I would like to state some signs here for you to watch out for in your elderly loved ones:

- Do they ask the same questions over and over?
- Do they act unusually or inappropriately?

- Do they get lost in places they know well?

- Do they forget recent events?

- Have you noticed changes in their personality?

- Are there changes in their eating habits or diet?

- Do they have recurrent falls or balance issues?

- Are there changes in their personal hygiene?

- Do they seem disinterested or indifferent about things they used to enjoy?

- Are they finding it hard to plan and organize tasks?

- Are there changes in their language skills, like how they understand things or the way they speak?

In conditions like Alzheimer's disease, these signs can sometimes become more noticeable, especially if something stressful or an illness pushes the brain beyond its ability to adapt. That's why regular check-ups are important since they help in tracking how cognitive abilities are changing and make sure that everyday independence is maintained as much as possible.

How Does the Brain Work?

The healthy human brain is made up of billions of special cells called neurons. These neurons send messages using electrical and chemical signals, helping different parts of the brain communicate with each other and with the rest of the body. In Alzheimer's disease, this communication gets disrupted, leading to a loss of brain function as many neurons stop working properly and ultimately die.[9]

Neurons have three main parts:

- *Cell Body:* This is where the nucleus is located. The nucleus acts like the brain of the neuron and directs and controls what the neuron does.

- *Dendrites:* These are branch-like extensions that come out from the cell body. They gather information from other neurons.

- *Axon:* This is a long, cable-like part that extends from the cell body and sends signals to other neurons.

Neurons are important for our brain, but they're not the only important cells. Glial cells, which support and protect neurons, are actually the most common type of cell in the brain. There are several types of glial cells, including microglia, astrocytes, and oligodendrocytes.

- *Microglia:* These cells act like the brain's cleanup crew and protect the neurons from damage and remove unwanted substances and debris.

- *Astrocytes:* Shaped like stars, these cells help with many tasks, including supporting neurons, regulating brain chemicals, and providing protection.

---

[9] National Institute on Aging. (n.d). *What happens in the brain in Alzheimer's disease.* U.S. Department of Health and Human Services. Retrieved September 11, 2024, from https://www.nia.nih.gov/health/alzheimers-causes-and-risk-factors/what-happens-brain-alzheimers-disease

- *Oligodendrocytes:* These cells create a protective layer called myelin around the axons of neurons, which helps them send electrical signals efficiently.

Glial cells also work closely with blood vessels in the brain and play a part in the brain's immune response. They help keep everything balanced so the brain works properly. Recent studies suggest that when microglia and astrocytes are activated, they might contribute to brain inflammation.[10]

As people age, their brains naturally shrink a bit, but they don't usually lose a lot of neurons. But in Alzheimer's disease, the damage is much more severe. Alzheimer's disease causes brain cells to slowly break down, which leads to memory loss, thinking problems, and changes in behavior. It is usually marked by two things in the brain: amyloid plaques and neurofibrillary tangles. Amyloid plaques are clumps of protein that build up between nerve cells, and neurofibrillary tangles are twisted strands of a protein called tau inside brain cells. These problems stop brain cells from talking to each other, and over time, the brain cells die, which leads to a decline in thinking and memory. Alzheimer's affects important brain functions like communication, digestion, and repair.

The disease first harms areas of the brain involved in memory, such as the entorhinal cortex and hippocampus. As it progresses, it also impacts parts of the brain that handle language, reasoning, and social behavior. Over time, Alzheimer's causes extensive damage, leading to a gradual loss of independence and, eventually, being lethal.

---

[10] See footnote 9.

Dementia – An Umbrella Term

Dementia is an umbrella term for a set of symptoms that affect memory and thinking skills. It's not just one disease but a way to describe different conditions that make it hard to remember things, think clearly, and interact with others that impact daily life.

The most well-known type of dementia is Alzheimer's disease (AD). With most types of dementia, symptoms slowly get worse over time because the nerve cells in the brain are being damaged. This gradual damage is called neurodegeneration and is a central part of how the disease progresses.

People with dementia can have a mix of symptoms, and what they experience depends on the type of dementia and which part of the brain is affected. These symptoms can also change as the disease affects more areas of the brain.

For instance, in Alzheimer's disease, early on, people might struggle with short-term memory because the brain area that helps with new memories is affected. Other common issues can include problems with speaking, organizing tasks, and finding their way around. You might also notice changes in their personality or them facing problems like depression, anxiety, or seeing things that aren't there. As dementia develops, these symptoms can become more noticeable and evolve over time.

A Spectrum of Dementias

The cause of dementia is not always clear. Scientists are still working to figure out what causes it, but they believe it has something to do with certain proteins building up in the brain and messing with how it works. Different types of dementia have different proteins involved. Each of these conditions has its own causes and symptoms, which makes understanding and managing dementia more complicated. For example, in Alzheimer's disease, there are proteins called beta-amyloid and tau. In Lewy body dementia, the protein alpha-synuclein is involved. Vascular dementia might be caused by changes in the brain's blood vessels.

Sometimes, dementia can be caused by something that can be treated, like a vitamin deficiency or a thyroid problem. Part of diagnosing dementia involves checking for these treatable causes to see if they might be affecting memory or thinking.

Let's have a look at the types of dementia to understand better.

Alzheimer's: The Most Common Form

As stated previously, the most well-known type of dementia is Alzheimer's disease (AD), which is responsible for a large number of cases. In 2020, about 5.8 million Americans were living with Alzheimer's. While younger people can develop the disease, it's rare. The risk of Alzheimer's increases as we age, with the number of people affected doubling every five years after the age of 65. By 2060, the number of people living with Alzheimer's is expected to rise to nearly 14 million.[11]

The symptoms of Alzheimer's can differ from person to person, but memory problems are often one of the first signs. Some people may also have difficulty finding the right words,

---

[11] Matthews, K. A., Xu, W., Gaglioti, A. H., Holt, J. B., Croft, J. B., Mack, D., & McGuire, L. C. (2019). Racial and ethnic estimates of Alzheimer's disease and related dementias in the United States (2015–2060) in adults aged≥ 65 years. *Alzheimer's & Dementia*, *15*(1), 17-24.

understanding visual images, or making good decisions early on. These issues with thinking and judgment can signal the beginning stages of the disease. As Alzheimer's progresses, symptoms tend to get worse and might lead to more confusion and noticeable changes in behavior.

Most people with Alzheimer's experience symptoms in their mid-60s or later. If the disease shows up before age 65, it's called early-onset Alzheimer's, which can start as early as someone's 30s, though this is quite rare.

Signs of Mild Alzheimer's Disease

When someone you love has mild Alzheimer's, they might still look healthy, but you may notice that things are getting harder for them. It's not always obvious right away, but over time, small changes begin to show, both to them and to you. Some things you might see are:

- They may be forgetting things that interrupt their daily life.

- They might make poor decisions or show poor judgment.

- They may seem less spontaneous or lose their usual initiative.

- They could get confused about dates or where they are.

- It might take them longer to finish everyday tasks.

- They may repeat questions or forget things they just learned.

- They could have trouble handling money or paying bills.

- They may struggle with planning or solving problems.

- They might wander off or get lost.

- They may lose things or put them in odd places.

- They might have difficulty with tasks like bathing or dressing.

- Their mood or personality could start to change.

- They may show signs of increased anxiety or even aggression.

It's often around this stage that Alzheimer's is diagnosed.

Signs of Moderate Alzheimer's Disease

At this stage, your loved one may need more supervision and care, which can be tough for spouses and families. You might notice changes like:

- They might be withdrawing themselves from social activities.

- They may struggle to learn new things.

- They could have trouble with language, reading, writing, or working with numbers.

- They might find it difficult to organize their thoughts or think logically.

- They may have a shorter attention span.

- They could struggle with new situations.

- They might experience changes in sleep patterns, like sleeping more during the day and being restless at night.

- They may have difficulty completing normal tasks with multiple steps, like getting dressed.

- They could occasionally have trouble recognizing family and friends.

- They might experience hallucinations, delusions, or paranoia.

- They may act impulsively, like undressing at inappropriate times or using vulgar language.

- They might have inappropriate emotional outbursts.

- They could become fidgety, agitated, anxious, tearful, or wander, especially later in the day.

- They may repeat statements or movements and have occasional muscle twitches.

These changes can be tough, but knowing what to expect can help you better support your loved one.

Signs of Severe Alzheimer's Disease

At this stage, your loved one will need complete care and won't be able to communicate. As their body begins to shut down, they may spend most or all of their time in bed. You might notice things like:

- They may not be able to communicate at all.

- They might have no awareness of recent experiences or their surroundings.

- They may lose weight and show little interest in eating.

- They could experience seizures.

- Their overall physical health may decline, including dental, skin, and foot problems.

- They might have trouble swallowing.

- You may hear them groaning, moaning, or grunting.

- They may sleep much more than usual.

- They could lose control of their bowel and bladder.

One common cause of death in people with severe Alzheimer's is aspiration pneumonia. This happens when they can't swallow properly, and food or liquids end up in their lungs rather than air.

Vascular Dementia

Vascular dementia is the second most common type of dementia and happens when the brain doesn't get enough oxygen because of reduced blood flow. Stroke is a major cause, and depending on which parts of the brain are affected, the symptoms can look different for everyone.

After a major stroke, you might notice things like confusion, trouble speaking or understanding speech, and even vision loss. Memory might not be the main problem, but you may see sudden changes in how your elderly loved one thinks or reasons. If there have been many small strokes, the changes can happen more slowly over time.

If your loved one has vascular dementia, you might notice signs like:

- They may have stroke-like symptoms, such as trouble in speaking.

- They could get easily confused or upset, especially at night.

- Their personality or mood might start to change.

- They may walk differently, like shuffling instead of lifting their feet.

- They might have poor balance.

- They could feel an urgent need to pee more often.

Unlike Alzheimer's, which usually begins with memory problems, vascular dementia might show up as trouble with planning, organizing, or making decisions.

Lewy Body Dementia

If your loved one has Lewy body dementia (LBD), it's caused by abnormal deposits of a protein called alpha-synuclein in the brain. This type of dementia makes up about 5% to 15% of all cases.[12]

There are some unique signs associated with LBD, such as fluctuating cognitive impairment with variations in attention and alertness, which basically means that they may have moments where their attention and alertness change a lot. One minute, they're focused, and the next, they might seem confused or out of it. They could also have complex visual hallucinations, where they could tell you of seeing things that aren't really there. They might also show signs of Parkinson's, like stiff movements or tremors, without having Parkinson's disease itself.[13] These symptoms can come and go, so it's important to pay attention to these changes over time.

---

[12] Duong, S., Patel, T., & Chang, F. (2017). Dementia: What pharmacists need to know. *Canadian Pharmacists Journal/Revue des Pharmaciens du Canada, 150*(2), 118-129.

[13] Zupancic, M., Mahajan, A., & Handa, K. (2011). Dementia with Lewy bodies: diagnosis and management for primary care providers. *The primary care companion for CNS disorders, 13*(5), 26212.

Along with this, you might notice fluctuations in their mental state as well. In fact, this happens in 30% to 89% of people with LBD. Unlike Alzheimer's, LBD often comes with changes where they might seem lethargic or unusually tired during the day, or they could have periods where they just stare blankly into space and not really engage with what's around them. There may be times when their memory suddenly seems to improve, or they might have episodes where their speech is disorganized or hard to follow. Their attention could come and go, sometimes being sharp and at other times much less focused.

Moreover, you may notice certain physical changes early on, such as muscle stiffness (rigidity) and slow movements (bradykinesia). They may also have rapid eye movement (REM) sleep disorders, like acting out their dreams. Even though memory loss is usually an early sign of Alzheimer's, it usually shows up later in LBD. In fact, more than 80% of people with LBD sooner or later develop Parkinson's-like symptoms, known as parkinsonism.

It's important to understand the difference between LBD and Parkinson's disease dementia (PDD). In LBD, dementia typically starts up to 12 months before any Parkinson's-like symptoms appear. With PDD, those Parkinson's symptoms, like tremors, usually show up around the same time as dementia.

In LBD, you're more likely to notice issues like postural instability and problems in walking, while tremors are more common in PDD.[14]

---

[14] Muangpaisan, W. (2007). Clinical differences among four common dementia syndromes. *Geriatrics and Aging, 10*(7), 425-429.

Frontotemporal Dementia

Frontotemporal dementia is a term for disorders that impact the frontal and temporal lobes of the brain, like Pick's disease.[15] It usually starts at a younger age (between 40 and 75 years) compared to Alzheimer's disease (AD).

If your loved one has FTD, you might notice signs like:

- They may have changes in their personality or behave differently.

- They might suddenly act without inhibitions in social situations.

- They could have trouble finding the right words when speaking.

- They might experience movement issues, like shakiness, unsteady balance, or muscle spasms.

One thing to remember is that, unlike Alzheimer's, FTD doesn't usually affect their ability to understand visual or spatial information.

Why Is It Important to Understand These Types?

Well, to put it simply, understanding the different types of dementia can make a difference in how well your loved one is cared for. Getting an accurate diagnosis is very important because each type of dementia has its own signs and progresses differently. When your elderly's doctor identifies the exact type, they can create a care plan that fits your loved one's specific needs.

---

[15] See footnote 12.

Along with this, effective treatment also depends on knowing the type of dementia. Different types may respond better to certain medications or therapies. Once the type is identified, doctors can recommend treatments that are most likely to help your elderly loved one as well as yourself in taking proper care of them.

You can also get help with guessing or recognizing the potential challenges and plan ahead when you know which type of dementia your loved one has. For instance, if your loved one has Alzheimer's disease, you might notice they become more disoriented over time. On the other hand, if they have frontotemporal dementia, you might see changes in their behavior. When you know what to expect, you can prepare for and manage these challenges more appropriately.

Chapter 5: Preparing for Diagnosis

As a caregiver for your elderly loved ones, you might be wondering what signs to watch for. Earlier, we talked about some general symptoms; now, let's focus on the signs of dementia.

Early Warning Signs

As previously discussed, dementia happens when healthy brain cells start losing their connections and eventually die. While some brain cell loss is a normal part of aging, dementia leads to much more significant changes, which come with noticeable symptoms.

In the early stages of mild Alzheimer's, a person may still look healthy on the outside, but they start having trouble understanding and interacting with the world around them. These changes can be subtle at first, so it can take time for both the person and their family to realize something is wrong.

For your elderly loved one who is going through these changes, it might feel like small memory slips or moments of confusion, which they might dismiss as just part of getting older. Because it starts slowly, it can take a while to recognize that something more serious is happening.

Here are some signs to watch for, though they can vary from person to person:

Memory Loss, Poor Judgment, and Confusion:

You might notice that your loved one starts to forget important things, like appointments or where they put things. They could make decisions that don't seem wise, like giving away money or trusting the wrong people. Sometimes, they might get confused about where they are or what day it is, even if it's something they used to know well.

For example, one day, your elderly might come to you and say they forgot where they parked their car, even though they've parked it in the same spot for years. Or, they might leave the stove on after cooking, something they never used to do.

Difficulty with Language:

Conversations could become harder for them. They might struggle to find the right words, pause a lot, or mix up words. What you or others are saying can also be problematic for them. You may notice that reading and writing, which they might use to do easily, become difficult or frustrating.

For example, you might notice that your loved one is trying to tell you a story but keeps getting stuck and is not able to find the right words. They might say, "You know, that thing we use to eat soup," instead of "spoon." Or they might struggle to follow along with a conversation and just nod without really understanding what's being said.

Wandering and Getting Lost:

Your loved one might leave the house and wander around without a clear purpose, even in familiar areas like their own neighborhood. This can be especially concerning if they get lost or can't find their way back home, which can put them at risk.

Financial Problems:

Managing money might become a big issue. They could forget to pay bills or lose track of spending. They might also become more vulnerable to scams or make poor financial decisions, which could lead to problems with their finances.

Repetitive Behavior:

You might start noticing that they ask the same questions over and over, or they might repeat the same actions, like folding the same item of clothing multiple times. For example, your loved one might ask you the same question repeatedly, like "What time is dinner?" even though you've just answered it. This can be frustrating, but it's important to remember that they're not doing it on purpose.

Unusual Language Use:

Sometimes, they might use strange or made-up words to describe things. For example, they might call a toothbrush a "mouth stick" or refer to a watch as a "time bracelet." This can be confusing, but it's a sign that their brain is struggling to find the right words.

Slower Daily Tasks:

Simple tasks, like getting dressed or making a cup of tea, might start taking a lot longer than they used to. They may get stuck or forget steps, which can be annoying for them and for you as well.

Loss of Interest:

You might notice that they don't seem to care about activities or hobbies they used to love. Whether it's gardening or spending time with friends, they might lose interest and seem more withdrawn.

Hallucinations and Paranoia:

They may start seeing or hearing things that aren't there, like thinking they see a person in the room when no one is there. They might also become suspicious of others, thinking people are stealing from them or plotting against them, even when that's not the case.

Impulsive Actions:

Your loved one might start doing things without thinking them through, like suddenly leaving the house, buying unnecessary items, or saying things that are out of character. This can lead to situations that are hard to manage.

Emotional Changes:

You might notice that they become less sensitive to other people's feelings. They may seem more self-centered or not able to show empathy, which can be a big change from how they used to be.

Loss of Balance and Movement Issues:

Physical changes can also occur. They might start having trouble walking, standing up from a chair, or maintaining their balance. These issues can increase the risk of falls and other injuries, so it's something to keep a close eye on.

It's also important to keep in mind that people with intellectual and developmental disabilities can experience dementia as they age, too. It might be harder to notice the signs in them, so pay attention to any changes in their usual abilities and behaviors.

Trigger Signs for a Doctor's Visit

It's important to know when it's time to see a doctor. While some changes can be subtle and gradual, there are certain 'trigger signs' that should prompt an immediate visit to the doctor. These are specific symptoms or situations that are not really part of normal aging and may point to a more serious issue.

Here are some examples:

- If your loved one suddenly forgets the names of close family members or can't remember important events, like a recent holiday or a visit from a friend, this is a strong sign that they need to see a doctor. Memory lapses that go past simple forgetfulness, especially if they happen quickly, are a cause for concern.

- If your elderly suddenly struggle to do things they've always done, like making a cup of tea, getting dressed, or using the phone, it's a sign that something isn't right. The tasks that used to be second nature to them becoming confusing or impossible is a clear trigger sign.

- If your loved one starts getting lost in places they've known for years, this is a serious sign that should prompt an immediate visit to the doctor. This kind of disorientation is more than just a momentary lapse and could show a deeper issue.

- If your loved one suddenly becomes aggressive, irritable, or starts acting in ways that are out of character for them, and these changes put their safety or relationships at risk, it's time to get medical help.

- If your loved one starts seeing or hearing things that aren't there or believes in things that are clearly not true (like thinking someone is trying to harm them when there's no evidence of that), these are red flags. Hallucinations and delusions can be frightening for both the person experiencing them and their family and require immediate medical attention.

Remember, it's always better to be cautious. These trigger signs might seem like minor issues to some people, but they're actually signals that something more serious could be going on. If you notice any of these signs, don't wait. Contact your loved one's doctor as soon as possible to make sure they receive the care they need.

Preparing for a Doctor's Appointment

When you take your elderly loved one to the doctor, it can be helpful to have a simple plan in place. Whether you're seeing a new doctor or going back to the same one, a little preparation can make the visit smoother for yourself as well as your elderly loved one. Here are some tips to help you in making sure you and the doctor cover everything your loved one needs:

Make A List of Concerns and Prioritize Them

Write down what you want to talk about before the appointment. If your loved one is capable of handling this list, ask them to make it and consider thinking about if there is a new symptom they're worried about. Do they want to ask about getting a flu shot? Maybe they're wondering how a treatment is going to affect their daily life. If you or your loved one have several things to discuss, try to list them in order of importance. Be sure to talk about the most pressing issues at the start of the visit so they don't get missed.

Bring Medications and Important Information

Some doctors suggest you bring all the medications your loved one is taking in a bag to the appointment. This includes prescription drugs, over-the-counter meds, vitamins, and supplements. Others might prefer a list that includes the name and dose of each. Also, don't forget to take along the contact information of your other doctors and any medical records the doctor might not already have.

Starting With a New Doctor

Starting with a new doctor can leave you and your loved one a bit unsure but it's a great chance to set up good communication from the beginning.

First things first, in my opinion, your elderly loved one should introduce themselves. What I mean is that when they meet the doctor and office staff, let them know what they'd like to be called. For example, your loved one might say, "Hi, I'm Mrs. Martinez," or "Good morning, my name is Bob Smith. Please call me Bob."

Secondly, take a moment to learn how things run in the office. Ask about the best times to call and what days are usually the busiest. It's also helpful to know what to do in case of an emergency or if your loved one is in need of care when the office is closed.

Moreover, it's also important to tell the doctor about your loved one's past illnesses, surgeries, and any other conditions. Also, mention any other doctors they've seen. Some doctors might send you a medical history form ahead of time so you can fill it out at home, where it's easier to gather the needed information. If filling out the forms feels confusing, don't hesitate to ask for help.

Make sure to give the new doctor the names and contact information of any previous doctors, especially if they are from a different city. This might help the new doctor in requesting copies of your loved one's medical records. You'll likely need to sign a form that gives permission for those records to be shared.

Take Someone Trusted Along to The Appointment

You can take a family member or close friend to the doctor's office, especially when you're caring for an elderly loved one. You might feel a little supported by doing this. Before the visit, let them know what you hope to get out of the appointment. They can help remind you of the things you want to talk about if you forget and take notes during the visit. That way, it's easier to remember what the doctor says afterward.

While a little extra support can be good, it's important to make sure that your companion doesn't take over the visit. This is your loved one's time with the doctor. If there are personal matters to discuss, you might want to ask your companion to wait in the waiting room for part of the appointment. Your loved one should also use time alone with the doctor during the physical exam to talk about private concerns (if there are any).

Keep the Doctor Updated

Make sure to share any changes in your loved one's health since the last visit. If they've been to the emergency room or seen a specialist, mention that. Also, bring up any changes in appetite, weight, sleep, behavior, or energy levels, and let the doctor know if any new medications have been prescribed or if there are any side effects.

See And Hear

If your loved one wears glasses, make sure they bring them. If they use a hearing aid, make sure it's working properly, and let the doctor know if there are any issues with hearing or seeing clearly. You can say something like, "My mom's hearing makes it hard to catch everything you're saying. It can be helpful if you speak slowly and face her when you talk." This will help the doctor communicate more effectively.

What to Expect at the Appointment

When it comes to figuring out if your elderly loved one has dementia, a doctor will need to look at different things, like what skills they've lost and what they can still do. Nowadays, doctors also use newer tests, called biomarkers, to help diagnose Alzheimer's more accurately. The doctor might start by reviewing your loved one's medical history and symptoms. They might ask someone close to your loved one, like you, to describe what you've noticed as well.

Please keep in mind that there isn't just one test that can tell if someone has dementia. Your loved one will likely go through a series of tests to help the doctor understand what's happening and rule out other causes.

Here's what to expect when you visit the doctor:

Initial Assessment

This is the first step the doctor will take to see if your loved one might have dementia. It's a process of elimination since there's no single test that can confirm dementia. The doctor might use terms like "probable Alzheimer's" or "probable dementia" because it can take time to get a full diagnosis. Sometimes, they might refer your loved one to a specialist.

During this initial assessment, the doctor will ask about your loved one's medical history and perform both physical and mental exams.

Questions About Medical History

The doctor might ask both you and your loved one questions about symptoms, like how long they've been happening and if there are any past illnesses or family history of medical or mental health issues. Some of their questions might be:

What symptoms are you noticing? Can you describe them?

When did you first see these changes?

Is there a family history of similar conditions or psychiatric issues?

Mental Status Exam

The doctor may also do some mental or cognitive tests. These look at your loved one's sense of time, memory, and ability to express themselves. It could include simple tasks like remembering words, drawing shapes, or answering questions like, "What year is it?" One common test is called the Montreal Cognitive Assessment (MoCA), which looks at things like judgment, memory, and problem-solving.

Physical Exam

To rule out other possible causes, the doctor might perform a physical exam and pay close attention to the brain and nervous system during it. They'll also check things like blood pressure, heart, and lungs, which can affect brain function. The doctor might also assess muscle strength, coordination, eye movement, speech, and sensation to get a better picture of what might be going on.

Supplementary Examinations

After the initial assessment, the doctor might have enough information to give a diagnosis. But if they need more details to be sure, they may recommend additional tests. These tests take more time, but they help in making the diagnosis as accurate as possible.

Your loved one might need detailed blood work. These tests help in checking for things like anemia, diabetes, or thyroid problems, which can sometimes add to dementia-like symptoms. The doctor may also order brain scans to look for signs of recent strokes or changes in blood vessels, like bleeding. Some tests that could be used include:

- CT or MRI scans, which take pictures of the brain's structure. This scan shows any shrinkage or other physical changes.

- SPECT scan, which shows how well blood is flowing through the brain.

- PET scan, which shows how different areas of the brain respond during activities like reading or talking. It usually involves resting for about 45 minutes before the scan.

- Sometimes, doctors can ask for sleep tests to be done to measure brain activity and see how well your loved one's brain is functioning.

Recommendation Of a Specialist

Your doctor might suggest that your loved one see a specialist or visit a memory clinic for further testing. If they don't bring it up and you think it would be helpful, you can always ask for a referral.

Specialists can be really helpful in diagnosing dementia.

The specialists your loved one might see include psychologists, psychiatrists, neurologists, geriatricians, nurses, social workers, or occupational therapists. They'll look closely at memory, reasoning, language, and judgment and how these things affect everyday life.

For example, a neurologist focuses on brain and nerve issues, a geriatrician specializes in elderly care, and a psychiatrist can help rule out other conditions like depression. If your doctor doesn't mention a referral and you feel it's necessary, don't hesitate to ask.

Please remember that specialists may overlap in their expertise, but they bring different perspectives to the table to assist in getting a more complete understanding of what's going on with your elderly.

Questions to Ask the Doctor

It's really important to work closely with the doctor and the health care team of your elderly loved one to create the best treatment plan for them. As Alzheimer's disease progresses, the goals of treatment are most likely going to change, so it's a good idea to understand all the options, along with the benefits and risks of each one.

When talking with the doctor about treatments, here are some questions that you can ask them:

- What treatment options are available?
- Is my loved one eligible for medications that can slow the disease?
- How will this drug help, and what changes might we see in daily life?
- Which symptoms do each medication target?
- How will we know if the treatment is working, and how long will it take?
- What side effects should we watch for at home, and how likely are they?

- If side effects happen, will we need to stop the medication?

- When should we call you about side effects or concerns?

- Will any treatments interfere with medications for other health issues?

- What happens if we need to switch from one medication to another?

- When would you recommend stopping a certain medication?

Some more questions that you can ask your elderly's doctor are:

- How can I help them remember things around the house?

- What's the best way to talk to them about memory loss?

- Should I use specific words or phrases when speaking to them?

- How should I ask questions or give instructions to them?

- Are there easier types of clothes or shoes they can wear to make dressing simpler?

- Can an occupational therapist help teach us new skills?

- What can I do to calm them down if they get confused or upset?

- Are there certain activities that might make them more agitated?

- How can I adjust the home to keep things calmer and safer for them?

- What should I do if they start wandering around?

- How can I keep them safe when they wander or try to leave the house?

- How do I make the house safer, i.e., what should I hide or put away?

- Should I make changes in the bathroom or kitchen to avoid accidents?

- Can they still manage their medications on their own?

- When should I start worrying about their driving being unsafe?

- How frequently should they get their driving assessed?

- What should I do if they refuse to stop driving?

- What kind of diet should I give them?

- Are there things I should watch for while they eat to prevent choking?

- What should I do if they do start choking?

I understand that caring for an elderly loved one with a condition such as this is not easy. But at this point, we can hope for a better outcome out of their condition and do things to make their life as comfortable as possible.

Chapter 6: The Misdiagnosis Challenge

If your loved one has been forgetting appointments or struggling to find the right words, it's natural to worry that it might be dementia or Alzheimer's. But did you know there are many other reasons why someone might be forgetful or make poor decisions? It's important to remember that there are many conditions that can cause similar symptoms, and many of them are treatable. Let's keep an open mind and think about all the possibilities. That way, they can get the help they need.

Sometimes, what looks like dementia in elderly patients might actually be a different condition called hepatic encephalopathy (HE), which is linked to liver problems like cirrhosis. It's important for you to know about this because, according to new research, patients with dementia should be screened for cirrhosis using a simple test called the Fibrosis-4 (FIB-4) index.

In a study involving over 68,000 people diagnosed with dementia between 2009 and 2019, almost 13% had FIB-4 scores that suggested cirrhosis and possible HE.[16] This means that quite a few people who are thought to have dementia may actually have a treatable condition related to liver function or something else.

---

[16] Silvey, S., Sterling, R. K., French, E., Godschalk, M., Gentili, A., Patel, N., & Bajaj, J. S. (2024). A Possible Reversible Cause of Cognitive Impairment: Undiagnosed Cirrhosis and Potential Hepatic Encephalopathy in Patients with Dementia. *The American Journal of Medicine*.

Dr. Jasmohan Bajaj, a researcher from Virginia Commonwealth University, highlighted that cirrhosis and related brain complications are common but usually go unnoticed, and they can be treated if detected early.[17] It's also worth noting that cirrhosis can lead to more serious issues like liver cancer, so it's important to diagnose it, even if dementia is suspected. So, understanding this link can make a big difference in getting the right treatment for your loved ones.

As I said, not all forgetfulness means dementia. There are other reasons, like delirium, normal pressure hydrocephalus, or mild cognitive impairment, that can also cause memory problems.

For example, frontotemporal dementia (FTD) can easily be mistaken for Alzheimer's disease (AD) or other conditions. Let's look at how they are different so you can understand what might be happening with your loved one.

Frontotemporal Dementia vs. Alzheimer's Disease

Since Alzheimer's is the most common type of dementia in older people, doctors often think of it first. But there are some key differences:

- *Age:* Alzheimer's becomes more common as people get older. Nonetheless, FTD usually starts earlier, typically in middle age.

---

[17] Larkin, M. (2024). Treatable condition misdiagnosed as dementia in almost 13% of cases. *Medscape.*
https://www.medscape.com/viewarticle/treatable-condition-misdiagnosed-dementia-almost-13-cases-2024a1000dif

- *Symptoms:* FTD usually starts with changes in behavior. Maybe your loved one is acting inappropriately, becoming more impulsive, or losing interest in things. People with early Alzheimer's have a tendency to still act socially appropriate and might even hide their memory problems well.

- *Apathy:* While people with Alzheimer's might show some lack of interest, it's usually mild. In FTD, the lack of concern can be much stronger - they may not care about others or show any desire to do things.

- *Memory vs. Behavior:* Alzheimer's usually starts with memory problems. Your loved one may have trouble remembering new information and later, even older memories start to fade. With FTD, memory problems aren't the main issue at first. They may still know the day, time, and place, but their behavior changes a lot more.

Frontotemporal Dementia vs. Psychiatric Disorders

Frontotemporal dementia (FTD) can also be mistaken for psychiatric disorders, especially when behavior changes are the main symptoms. Let's break down how this can happen:

- *Age Matters:* If FTD starts in middle age, it might look like late-life depression. If it starts earlier, it can be confused with conditions like schizophrenia or bipolar disorder.

- *Repetitive Behaviors:* People with a type of FTD called behavioral variant FTD (bvFTD) usually show repetitive, compulsive actions, which can lead to a diagnosis of obsessive-compulsive disorder (OCD) at first.

Because the behavior of someone with FTD can look a lot like that of someone with a psychiatric disorder, doctors usually need more information to make the right diagnosis. Neuropsychological tests, which measure memory and other skills, and brain imaging like an MRI are very helpful. An MRI can rule out other diseases and support the FTD diagnosis.

Diagnosing Frontotemporal Dementia

To diagnose FTD, doctors start by ruling out other possibilities. They'll look at:

- *Medical Exam and Personal History:* Information from the patient, family, or caregivers helps to understand the symptoms and changes over time.

- *Neuropsychological Tests:* These tests measure memory, language, and thinking skills to identify any specific issues.

- *Brain Imaging:* MRI scans are commonly used, but sometimes doctors may use other scans, like a PET scan, to see areas of the brain that are more or less active. This helps confirm an FTD diagnosis, especially in the frontal and temporal areas of the brain.

It Might Not Be Alzheimer's

While the number of Americans with Alzheimer's is expected to rise from 5 million to 16 million by 2050, research shows that about 1 in 5 Alzheimer's cases may actually be misdiagnosed. As Dr. Marc Agronin, a geriatric psychiatrist, points out, diagnosing Alzheimer's can be complicated. [18] It is

---

[18] HumanGood. (n.d.). *Top five dementia misdiagnoses.* HumanGood.

important to note that not all doctors have the right tools or experience to make the correct diagnosis.

Sometimes, people who have mild memory changes and feel confused don't have Alzheimer's at all. Here are five common conditions that are often mistaken for Alzheimer's:

1. Other Neurocognitive Disorders

Alzheimer's is the most well-known cause of memory problems, but it's not the only one. There are other types of dementia and medical issues that affect mental abilities, like vascular dementia or Parkinson's disease. For example, if a senior has a small stroke or even a benign brain growth, they could show signs of memory trouble.

Dr. Agronin shares a story about one of his patients who was quickly getting worse. The doctor assumed it was Alzheimer's and didn't even do a brain scan. It turned out that the patient had a large, non-cancerous tumor. Once it was removed, the patient lived another ten years.

2. Mild Cognitive Impairment (MCI)

If you've noticed your loved one struggling with short-term memory, like forgetting what they did earlier in the day, it could be a sign of Mild Cognitive Impairment (MCI). But the thing is that memory problems don't always mean it's Alzheimer's. Sometimes, it's just part of getting older, like forgetting names or phone numbers. It's important to pay attention to how these memory issues affect their daily life. If they can still manage on their own and the memory lapses are

https://www.humangood.org/resources/senior-living-blog/top-five-dementia-misdiagnoses

minor, that's pretty normal with age. However, if the memory problems are starting to interfere with daily tasks or independence, that's a good reason to talk to their doctor. They can help figure out if it's just part of aging or something else like MCI.

3. <u>Bipolar & Mood Disorders</u>

Now, if you notice your loved one showing other symptoms, like being really agitated or struggling with focus, it could be more than just memory issues. These could be signs of mood disorders like bipolar disorder. Mood disorders can make it hard to remember things or focus on tasks, and that can sometimes be mistaken for memory loss related to Alzheimer's. But again, it might not be dementia at all. In this case, it's best to see a neurologist or a doctor to get a proper diagnosis. They'll help you figure out if it's a mood disorder or something else like dementia so you can get the right care for your elderly.

4. <u>Delirium</u>

Sometimes, things like infections, surgeries, or even new medications can cause delirium, which can turn out to be really confusing for both you and your loved one. They might seem anxious, restless, or even depressed, and they could have trouble speaking or understanding speech. This might look a lot like dementia or Alzheimer's, but it might just be delirium. Before jumping to conclusions, it's important to take a look at any new medications they've started. Some medicines can cause these symptoms, so a doctor might suggest switching them to something else. If they're showing signs of confusion or memory issues, it could also be related to an infection or another health problem. That's why it's important to have a doctor check them out to see if it's delirium or something else.

5. Normal Pressure Hydrocephalus (NPH)

NPH is a condition where fluid builds up in the brain and creates pressure. This pressure can damage brain tissue and lead to symptoms that seem a lot like Alzheimer's, like disorientation or confusion. If your loved one is showing signs of forgetfulness or confusion, it might not be Alzheimer's at all - it could be NPH. The only way to know for sure is to see a doctor who can do tests to find out if NPH is the cause.

6. Vitamin B-12 Deficiency

As people get older, they sometimes don't eat as much or skip meals, which can lead to vitamin deficiencies. One of the most important vitamins for brain function is B-12, and if your loved one isn't getting enough of it, they could experience memory loss, depression, or even behavior changes. Sometimes, this can look a lot like dementia, but it's actually just a lack of B-12. If you notice any of these symptoms, it's a good idea to have their doctor check for a vitamin deficiency. It's an easy fix once it's caught, and they might get back to feeling like themselves again with the right treatment.

7. Alcohol and Memory Loss

If your loved one has been drinking heavily for a long time, this could be one reason for memory problems. Too much alcohol can damage brain cells and make memory issues worse. It can also lead to accidents or increase the risk of other health conditions, like liver disease, which can also affect how the brain works.

8. Medications and Cognition

Medications, whether they're prescribed or bought over the counter, can sometimes mess with memory and thinking.

Older adults, in particular, are more sensitive to these side effects. Plus, many seniors take multiple medications at once, which can lead to confusion or memory problems due to how the drugs interact with each other. This is why it's super important to let all of their doctors and pharmacists know what medications they're on. They can help spot if any of the meds are causing issues and make adjustments if needed.

9. Other Common Causes of Memory Loss

There are other things that can cause memory problems, too, like infections (especially urinary tract infections), thyroid issues, or even hearing and vision problems. If you're seeing memory issues, the best thing to do is get it checked out by a specialist.

Just like how you wouldn't go to a foot doctor for a heart problem, it's important to see the right kind of specialist for memory issues. They can help piece together what's really going on and figure out if it's Alzheimer's, another condition, or something else entirely.

Importance of Seeking a Doctor's Evaluation

If someone is wrongly diagnosed with dementia, it can cause a lot of unnecessary stress. Can you imagine being told you have dementia when you don't? Well, it's scary! Plus, they might end up with treatments they don't need, which can be frustrating and very overwhelming. It can also mean using healthcare services that aren't helpful, which might affect everyone. That's why making sure the diagnosis is correct is really important for the health of your elderly loved ones.

In my opinion, the best way to avoid misdiagnosis is to have a team of different healthcare experts working together, which could include doctors, nurses, pharmacists, and therapists. When all of these people talk to each other and share what they know, it's easier to spot what's really going on. Sometimes, mistakes happen because there isn't enough communication between the healthcare team, the patient, and their family. But if everyone works together, it's more likely your loved one will get the right diagnosis and care.

If your loved one is misdiagnosed, it can affect more than just their health. It could lead to legal issues about whether they can make decisions for themselves. This is why it's so important for everyone - family, caregivers, and healthcare professionals - to speak up if something doesn't seem right. Asking questions and sharing concerns can help protect your loved one's rights and make sure they get the right care.

So, if you're noticing signs of memory loss or confusion in your loved one, the best thing to do is to see a doctor who can really take the time to figure out what's going on. The right diagnosis means the right care and peace of mind for everyone.

Importance of Early Diagnosis

You or your loved one might be thinking, "Are my symptoms really bad enough to see a doctor?" That's totally normal, but getting checked out sooner rather than later can make a big difference. In fact, a lot of people with dementia say they wish they had gotten diagnosed earlier. I think it's not just about knowing what's going on but more about getting the right support when it is needed.

While there's no cure for dementia yet, there's a lot of support available to help your loved one live as well as possible. Getting diagnosed early helps you understand what kind of dementia it is and opens doors to support groups, therapies, and even medicines that can help manage symptoms. This support can help and might make things a little easier for your loved one as well as yourself as their caregiver.

Also, note that a dementia diagnosis means your loved one might be entitled to financial benefits. Plus, it legally protects them from being treated unfairly because of their condition. Having a clear diagnosis can help in making sure your loved one is getting the rights and help they deserve.

Yes, it can be frustrating when others don't understand why things are becoming harder for your elderly. A diagnosis can help explain those changes to the people around them and make it easier for them to support your loved one in the right way.

So, if you've noticed changes, don't brush them off as "not important." You and your loved one deserve to know what's going on, and healthcare professionals are there to help.

Is There a Cure for Dementia?

I can understand that it can be really hard when you're caring for someone with dementia and you're wondering if there's a cure. Right now, there isn't a cure for dementia, and that's because it's not just one disease. As we discussed, Dementia can be caused by different conditions, like Alzheimer's or frontotemporal dementia. So, finding one single cure is tough.

But the good news is that the researchers are making a lot of progress. They're working really hard to understand what exactly is happening in the brain to cause dementia. They're also looking for ways to stop or slow it down. Even though a full cure might still be a few years away, there are some exciting advancements being made.

Stem Cells

For example, scientists are using something called stem cells, which are special cells that can grow into different kinds of cells, like brain cells. They've found a way to take skin cells from people with certain types of dementia and turn them into brain cells in the lab. This helps them study how the brain gets damaged and what might help in stopping it. These brain cells are also used to test new treatments before trying them on real people.

Immunotherapy

Immunotherapy is a new approach that researchers are looking into to help fight dementia. It works by boosting the body's own immune system, similar to how it's been used to treat diseases like cancer.

In dementia, some treatments being studied focus on abnormal proteins that build up in the brain, especially in Alzheimer's disease. For example, scientists have tried creating a vaccine to target these proteins. Another treatment they're exploring involves using something called 'monoclonal antibodies,' which are like man-made versions of what the immune system naturally produces. These antibodies aim to attack the harmful proteins and slow the disease. Some of these trials have had mixed results, but a few have shown potential and are being considered as possible treatments.

Another area being studied is the brain's own immune cells, called *microglia*. These cells help in clearing out waste in the brain. But in Alzheimer's disease, they can become too active and may start causing more damage than good. Researchers are trying to figure out how to prevent this from happening.

Gene-based Therapies

There's also a lot of excitement around gene-based therapies. These focus on targeting specific genes that might lead to dementia, like those involved in Alzheimer's or frontotemporal dementia. Some of these therapies are also being used to reduce the production of harmful proteins in the brain.

Repurposing Medicines

Creating new medicines for dementia can take a long time and cost a lot of money. So, scientists are also trying a quicker way by using medicines that already exist for other health problems. These are medicines for things like type 2 diabetes, high blood pressure, or even erectile dysfunction.

Since these medicines are already used safely for other conditions, researchers are now testing them to see if they can help people with Alzheimer's or vascular dementia. This might help in finding treatments for dementia more quickly than starting from scratch.

You Can Join the Research!

There are many dementia research projects happening worldwide. If you or a loved one has been diagnosed with dementia or you're noticing memory problems, you can join these studies! You can help the scientists discover more about the disease and work toward future treatments.

And it's not just for those with dementia. If you're a caregiver, your role is just as important! There are research projects focused on finding the best ways to care for someone with dementia, and your input could help in improving care for families just like yours!

Chapter 7: The Road Ahead

When you're caring for someone with dementia, it's natural to hope for a cure. But as we discussed earlier, right now, there isn't one. I can understand that it can be hard to hear this and it might feel devastating too. But while there's no single solution to stop the progression of dementia, there are some ways to make life a little better - for both the person living with dementia and the people around them. We discussed some of the advancements made by researchers before, and I would like to touch base on some treatment approaches here. From medications to therapies, you can say that there is support out there. These treatments, or you can say approaches, might not take the disease away, but they might make the road ahead a little smoother.

Medications

While a cure doesn't seem to be available right now, there are four medications approved by Health Canada that may help manage some of the symptoms.[19] These can assist with things like changes in language, thinking, and movement, and they might make a difference in day-to-day life. These medications usually come in both brand-name and generic names:

- Aricept™ (Donepezil)

---

[19] Alzheimer Society of Canada. (n.d.). *Medications approved for Dementia in Canada*. Alzheimer Society of Canada. Retrieved October 23, 2024, from https://alzheimer.ca/en/about-dementia/dementia-treatment-options-developments/medications-for-alzheimers

- Reminyl ER™ (Galantamine)

- Exelon™ (Rivastigmine)

- Ebixa® (Memantine)

It doesn't really matter if you choose the brand-name or generic since they work the same way and can help make things a bit easier. Figuring out which medication is right can depend on how severe the symptoms are and how quickly the disease is progressing. Different medications may be appropriate at different stages.

Cholinesterase inhibitors - like donepezil, galantamine, and rivastigmine - were originally created to treat Alzheimer's disease. While they weren't developed for other types of dementia or conditions like mild cognitive impairment, these medications are now usually used for various types of dementia, with the exception of frontotemporal dementia. That said, since each form of dementia may come with its own treatment recommendations, it's always a good idea to discuss the options with your doctor.

For those in the early stages of Alzheimer's, treatments like donepezil, galantamine, or rivastigmine are usually prescribed to help manage the symptoms. As the disease progresses to moderate or advanced stages, medications like memantine or higher doses of donepezil may be recommended. When it comes to Lewy body dementia, a combination of donepezil, galantamine, rivastigmine, and memantine may be used to help ease the symptoms and slow the development.

For people living with Parkinson's disease dementia, rivastigmine is generally the most commonly prescribed option. While these treatments can't stop the disease, they are designed to make daily life more manageable by taking into consideration specific symptoms. As always, it's important to regularly review any treatment plan with your elderly's doctor to make sure it's personalized to your loved one's changing needs.

I understand it can be too much to sort through different treatment options, especially when it comes to explicit types of dementia. For people living with vascular dementia or frontotemporal dementia, there isn't enough evidence to support the use of cholinesterase inhibitors or memantine. These medications aren't generally recommended for those conditions.

But, if someone has a combination of Alzheimer's disease and vascular dementia, referred to as mixed dementia, cholinesterase inhibitors may be used if Alzheimer's is the main cause of the symptoms. It's important to note here that these medications won't treat vascular dementia on their own, but they can help if Alzheimer's is part of the picture.

For mild cognitive impairment, these treatments aren't usually effective either. They don't seem to reduce the chances of MCI progressing into Alzheimer's disease or another type of dementia, so they're generally not recommended in these cases.

It's also important to remember that dementia affects everyone differently. A treatment that works well for one person might not work the same way for someone else.

How Do These Medications Work?

You might be wondering how these medications actually work to help with memory and learning. Three of the most commonly used medications - donepezil (Aricept™), galantamine (Reminyl™), and rivastigmine (Exelon™) - are known as cholinesterase inhibitors. What they do is help prevent the breakdown of a brain chemical called acetylcholine, which plays an important role in learning and memory.

To explain a bit more about acetylcholine, it's a chemical in the brain that helps with communication between nerve cells. In someone with Alzheimer's disease, the levels of acetylcholine are much lower than in a person without the disease. These medications work by increasing the concentration of acetylcholine in the brain, which may help temporarily ease or stabilize some of the symptoms of dementia. This isn't a cure, but it can make a difference in managing memory loss and cognitive decline for a while.

Typically, these medications might be effective for around two to three years, possibly longer in some cases. However, as the disease grows and nerve endings in the brain eventually die, the medications stop working. This is why they're usually prescribed for people in the mild to moderate stages of dementia when they might still offer some benefit.

You might also want to know how medications like memantine (Ebixa®) work. It is said that memantine might help protect brain cells. Memantine is different from the cholinesterase inhibitors we've discussed - it's an NMDA receptor antagonist. This medication works by influencing another brain chemical called glutamate, which plays a role in sending messages between brain cells.

In someone with Alzheimer's disease, glutamate can overstimulate the NMDA receptors, which can cause damage to nerve cells. Memantine helps by blocking the effects of too much glutamate and protecting the brain cells from further harm. This makes it a useful option for people in the middle to later stages of Alzheimer's, especially for those who may not tolerate the side effects of cholinesterase inhibitors.

Some specialists even recommend using memantine and cholinesterase inhibitors together to get the benefits of both.

Nevertheless, more research is needed to confirm the efficacy of this combination.

You might also wonder how you can tell if a medication is really making a difference. It's important to know that improvements might be subtle, and it might take a few months before you notice any changes. Even for doctors and pharmacists, these improvements can be hard to detect right away, as the benefits may vary from person to person.

When a medication is working, you might notice small cognitive improvements, such as better memory, concentration, or language skills. There could also be subtle behavioral changes. For instance, your loved one might become calmer, more engaged in daily activities like cooking or bathing, or more communicative and motivated. Some people may not have big changes but could stay stable for a while, which can also be considered a good outcome. For example, if your loved one used to forget simple things, they might start remembering them again, or if they were restless, they might now feel more peaceful.

Possible Side Effects

It's important to remember that medications are usually given in small doses at first to reduce side effects. If the person responds well to a medication, the doctor may slowly increase the amount to get the most benefit from the treatment. For example, someone may start with a low dose and have it adjusted over time to find what works best for them while minimizing any negative effects.

You might want to talk to your loved one's doctor to get a full list of possible side effects specific to the medication they're taking. If any of the side effects do occur, don't hesitate to reach out to the doctor or pharmacist.

Here are some potential side effects of common medications like donepezil, galantamine, and rivastigmine:

- Gastrointestinal issues, such as nausea, vomiting, diarrhea, or loose stools

- Loss of appetite, which might lead to unintended weight loss

- A slowing heart rate

- Dizziness or even falls

- Headaches

- Nightmares or other sleep disruptions

It's worth noting that sleep issues, like insomnia, can sometimes depend on when the medication is taken. For example, some experts recommend taking donepezil (Aricept) in the morning to help avoid sleep disturbances at night.

Now, let's look at some possible side effects of memantine:

- Feeling drowsy or sleepy (sedation)

- Muscle cramps

- Headaches

- Dizziness

- Feeling tired or fatigued

- Trouble sleeping (insomnia)

Just like with the other medications, sleep problems can sometimes be a side effect. Make sure to talk to the doctor or pharmacist if the person you're caring for is having trouble sleeping or if you're unsure about the timing of the medication.

Also, if your elderly loved one has any kidney problems, extra care might be needed when prescribing memantine. Be sure to discuss this with the doctor.

No Changes Can Be a Good Thing

Alzheimer's and other forms of dementia are progressive diseases, which means they get worse over time. So, if you don't notice any changes in your loved one's daily activities or behavior for six months to a year after starting the medication, that might actually be a positive thing. It means the medication may be working to help slow the progression.

But, if the medication is stopped, the person might lose those benefits and could decline more quickly than expected. That's why it's important to talk with your loved one's healthcare team before making any changes to the treatment plan.

When Should These Medicines Be Started?

If there aren't any other health conditions that could make these medications unsafe for your loved one, doctors usually recommend starting a trial as soon as a person is diagnosed with dementia. Starting early might give the medication the best chance to help.

If your elderly's doctor seems unsure or doesn't want to prescribe one of these medications, it might be a good idea to ask for a second opinion from a geriatric specialist. They have more experience working with dementia treatments and might provide you with a different perspective.

Now, you might ask that for how long should your loved one take these medications. Well, if you find that the medication is helping and the side effects aren't too difficult to manage, it's usually suggested to keep taking it throughout the course of the disease, even into the later stages.

On the other hand, if the medication doesn't seem to be making a noticeable difference, causes too many side effects, or if your loved one or you simply don't feel comfortable about it, it may be time to consider stopping. Remember, each person's experience is different. Discuss with your elderly's doctor what makes the most sense for your loved one.

Non-pharmacological Therapies

There are other ways to get help with dementia that don't involve taking medicine. It's important to pick options that are proven to work. These are normally called alternative treatments, and they don't use drugs. For example, some therapies can benefit your loved one by managing their stress and making them feel a bit better without the risk of side effects that come with medications. To understand better, you can think about things like exercise. These alternate treatments or approaches might help, but it's always a good idea to check if they're backed by research.

It's really worth thinking about alternative treatments for a few reasons. First, they give us hope for options that don't rely on medications and their risks. Second, they can bring positive changes in the quality of life for both your elderly loved one diagnosed with dementia and yourself by providing some much-needed relief. And finally, choosing treatments supported by research is important. It reassures us that we're using something proven to benefit.

Cognitive Stimulation Therapy

Cognitive Stimulation Therapy (CST) is an evidence-based, non-pharmacological method of treating complex behavioral and psychological symptoms in dementia patients.[20,21] Disruptive behaviors, mood swings, hallucinations, anger, anxiety, difficulty sleeping, motor changes, apathy, depression, loss of memory are all possible symptoms of BPSD.[22]

Behavioral and psychological symptoms of dementia (BPSD) can lead to negative consequences for patients, such as isolation, helplessness, and a higher risk of falls and injuries, which lower their quality of life. These symptoms can also increase stress for caregivers, which can contribute to burnout and higher hospitalization rates. Furthermore, BPSD usually results in the need for admission to skilled care facilities.[23]

Cognitive Stimulation Therapy (CST) is aimed to keep your loved one's brain active with engaging activities. Activities that stimulate the mind, like puzzles or discussions, can boost their thinking, focus, and memory. The idea is to work on skills that are still there, like 'implicit memory,' which is more

---

[20] YY Szeto, J., & JG Lewis, S. (2016). Current treatment options for Alzheimer's disease and Parkinson's disease dementia. *Current neuropharmacology, 14*(4), 326-338.

[21] Abraha, I., Rimland, J. M., Trotta, F. M., Dell'Aquila, G., Cruz-Jentoft, A., Petrovic, M., ... & Cherubini, A. (2017). Systematic review of systematic reviews of non-pharmacological interventions to treat behavioural disturbances in older patients with dementia. The SENATOR-OnTop series. *BMJ open, 7*(3), e012759.

[22] Ohno, Y., Kunisawa, N., & Shimizu, S. (2019). Antipsychotic treatment of behavioral and psychological symptoms of dementia (BPSD): management of extrapyramidal side effects. *Frontiers in pharmacology, 10*, 1045.

[23] Feast, A., Moniz-Cook, E., Stoner, C., Charlesworth, G., & Orrell, M. (2016). A systematic review of the relationship between behavioral and psychological symptoms (BPSD) and caregiver well-being. *International psychogeriatrics, 28*(11), 1761-1774.

automatic. So, while it may not feel like formal treatment, it's a gentle way to help them stay connected, engaged, and even feel a bit more confident.

(CST) was developed by Dr. Spector and her team in the UK. It's recognized by the National Institute for Health and Care Excellence (NICE) as a proven way to help manage mild to moderate dementia. CST focuses on improving confidence, thinking skills, social interaction, and overall life quality. It's an evidence-based approach, meaning it's been studied and shown to work, which can give you some peace of mind knowing that your loved one is getting effective, non-drug support.

A study by Saragih and colleagues from 2022 says that Cognitive Stimulation Therapy is something we should think about including in dementia care. It seems to benefit by improving thinking skills and might even lower depression in people with mild to moderate dementia.[24]

That said, more research is needed to see if CST also helps with some of the behavior changes that can come with dementia. Plus, we need more studies to figure out the best way to actually assess and use CST in a real, practical way.

You might be wondering how CST is actually done. Well, it's usually offered as a group therapy for people with dementia who are at similar stages cognitively. The whole idea is to make the activities fun, centered around the person, and mentally

---

[24] Saragih, I. D., Tonapa, S. I., Saragih, I. S., & Lee, B. O. (2022). Effects of cognitive stimulation therapy for people with dementia: A systematic review and meta-analysis of randomized controlled studies. *International Journal of Nursing Studies, 128*, 104181.

stimulating. Things that help with memory, reasoning, and language.

Typically, the group has about six to eight people, and it's run by two facilitators. The program lasts for about seven weeks, with two sessions each week, so that's 14 visits in total. Each week has a theme, and they cover a variety of topics from childhood memories to current events and even activities like baking or word games.

The sessions might start with a group welcome. They also use something called a reality orientation board, which might keep everyone on track and keep things consistent from one session to the next. I think the best part is that the participants get to suggest activities or themes, which makes it more personal and engaging for them.

CST can actually be offered in different places, like in the community or long-term care homes. There was even a study that looked at how CST works in a hospital setting. In this case, the researchers made some changes to the program for patients with dementia who were staying in the hospital.

They found that not only did patients and their caregivers enjoy it,[25] but there were some other positive effects too. For example, because the participants ate together during the sessions, their nutrition improved. Plus, since they had to leave their rooms to attend, their mobility got better, and they also became more social. Since hospital stays are usually short, the program was modified to fit that time frame, but the benefits were still clear.

---

[25] McAulay, J., & Streater, A. (2020). Delivery of cognitive stimulation therapy for people with dementia in an inpatient setting (innovative practice). *Dementia, 19*(7), 2513-2520.

Occupational Therapy

The main goal of occupational therapy (OT) for people with dementia is to improve their health and overall quality of life - and yours, too.

An occupational therapist will work closely with you and your loved one to figure out which tasks are becoming difficult. You could come up with strategies together to make those tasks safer and more manageable.

Occupational therapy of your loved one might help them maintain their independence and the therapist can also connect you with other services, organizations, and networks. They might give you advice on how to support your loved one in the best way possible.

The American Occupational Therapy Association (AOTA) highlights several ways that occupational therapy (OT) can help your elderly. One of the main things an Occupational therapist does is teach skills that make everyday activities, like bathing, dressing, and eating, easier. They also help with cognitive skills, things like concentration, memory, planning, and prioritizing. So, if your loved one is having trouble staying focused or remembering things, the OT can show them techniques to improve that.

The OT might also suggest adaptive equipment to help your loved one do more on their own. This could be special cutlery for easier eating, bathroom aids like handrails or shower seats, or even visual aids for getting dressed, like labels or photos to help them find the right clothes.

Safety at home is another area where an OT can step in. They might recommend things like grab rails, non-slip mats, better lighting, or clearing out clutter in order to prevent falls.

They could also suggest removing locks from doors so your loved one doesn't accidentally lock themselves in.

All in all, an OT can give you advice on how to better support your loved one as they go through life with dementia.

Behavioral Interventions

Behavioral interventions are about understanding and handling the difficult behaviors that usually come with dementia. These can include things like aggression, wandering, or agitation. These behaviors can be really hard on both your loved one and you as a caregiver. The goal is to figure out what's causing these behaviors and find ways to reduce or stop them.

One of the first steps in this approach is figuring out what triggers these behaviors. Usually, behaviors like agitation or aggression are prompted by something that's bothering your loved one. They might be uncomfortable, confused, or frustrated but can't communicate it the way they used to. For example, someone might get agitated because the environment is too noisy, or they might wander because they're feeling restless or trying to find something they're familiar with.

Another part of behavioral interventions is creating a supportive and calming environment. Sometimes, simplifying things around your loved one, like reducing clutter, turning down loud noises, or setting up a consistent daily routine might help in reducing their stress and confusion. This can make your elderly feel more comfortable, which in turn might make the behaviors less likely to occur.

Rather than focusing only on stopping the behavior, behavioral interventions also encourage positive behaviors. This means trying to shift their focus away from something that's upsetting them by gently guiding them toward something enjoyable or calming. For example, if they're upset, you could suggest going for a short walk to make them feel better.

Caregivers play an important role in this approach, too. You might be the one who notices when a behavior is starting and can use these techniques to respond. Learning to react in a calm, gentle way might reduce tension and make things easier for both of you.

Behavioral interventions might work best when used alongside other non-pharmacological approaches, like CST and OT.

Lifestyle Modifications

A recent study published in Alzheimer's Research & Therapy looked into how intensive lifestyle changes can help people in the early stages of Alzheimer's disease.[26] Over a 20-week period, researchers found that combining several healthy habits, like following a plant-based diet, exercising, managing stress, and attending group support meetings, could help improve mental function.

This means that lifestyle changes may not only help those already showing signs of dementia but might be considered as a way to prevent it from getting worse or might even stop it from developing. The study points to how important it is to

---

[26] Ornish, D., Madison, C., Kivipelto, M., Kemp, C., McCulloch, C. E., Galasko, D., ... & Arnold, S. E. (2024). Effects of intensive lifestyle changes on the progression of mild cognitive impairment or early dementia due to Alzheimer's disease: a randomized, controlled clinical trial. *Alzheimer's Research & Therapy, 16*(1), 122.

focus on healthy eating, staying active, and handling stress to support brain health.

Maintaining A Healthy Diet

You might have heard that what you eat affects your physical health. Well, I read that it might also have a big impact on your brain. There's now some evidence showing that the right diet might lower the chances of developing dementia while also being great for the heart.

It makes sense to take care of both the heart and the brain. Heart or circulatory diseases can increase a person's risk of dementia, so keeping the heart healthy can be considered as one way to help protect the brain too.

One diet that's been created to specifically target brain health is the MIND diet (Mediterranean-DASH Intervention for Neurodegenerative Delay). It was developed by researchers at Rush University in Chicago to help prevent dementia and slow down brain aging. The MIND diet combines two well-known, heart-healthy diets:

- The Mediterranean diet is rich in whole grains, fish, beans, fruits, and vegetables.

- The DASH diet (Dietary Approaches to Stop Hypertension) focuses on controlling blood pressure by reducing salt intake, which is another risk factor for heart disease and dementia.

Both of these diets have a lot of research behind them supporting their benefits for heart health. There's also some evidence that they might play a role in slowing down mental decline. The MIND diet specifically highlights some brain-boosting foods to eat regularly and suggests limiting five foods that may not be as good for cognitive function.

117

The brain boosting foods include wholegrains, suggested to have at least three servings a day. Green leafy vegetables like spinach, kale, and salad greens should also be part of the daily meals. Along with these, aim to eat and make your loved one eat other vegetables every day. Nuts are another brain-boosting food and are best eaten most days of the week. Beans and lentils, rich in nutrients, should be eaten at least three times a week. Berries, particularly blueberries and strawberries, are known for their brain benefits, so it's advised to try to eat them twice a week. Including chicken or turkey in the meals two or more times a week is another great way to support brain health. Fish is one more important food, and having it once a week might make a difference. Cooking with olive oil is encouraged, as it is a healthier fat choice.

On the flip side, there are some foods named by the MIND diet to avoid or limit to help the brain stay healthy. Fried or fast food should be kept to less than once a week. Cheese is also something to eat sparingly, ideally no more than once a week. Red meats can be eaten up to four times a week, but it's best to limit them. Pastries and sweets should be enjoyed less than five times a week, and butter should be limited to less than one tablespoon a day.

Regular Exercise

Exercise is another part of a healthy lifestyle. Regular physical activity benefits the body and it's good for the brain, too. Even light activities like walking or gentle stretching might improve your loved one's mood, increase their energy, and might even assist in maintaining their mobility. Exercise might also reduce restlessness and anxiety, which are common in dementia. Plus, being active can improve heart health, which is closely connected to brain function.

If your loved one enjoys certain physical activities, like gardening or swimming, encourage them to keep doing those. The important thing is to find something they enjoy so it doesn't feel like a chore.

Quality Sleep

Getting good sleep is really important for brain health. But with dementia, sleep can often be tricky. As mentioned earlier, your loved one might have trouble falling asleep or wake up a lot during the night. It's frustrating, but there are some simple things you can try to improve your elderly's sleep.

First, think about creating a calming bedtime routine. Something like a warm bath or reading a book can be soothing and help them wind down. You might also try sticking to a regular sleep schedule, even on weekends. If they're feeling restless at night, it might be worth looking at how much they're napping during the day. You can limit the naps and make sure they get enough sunlight and physical activity so that they sleep better at night.

Doctor Visits After Diagnosis

Regular follow-up appointments with the doctor after a dementia diagnosis are really important for keeping track of how things are going with your loved one's health. Dementia is a progressive condition, so these appointments might allow the doctor to monitor any changes in symptoms, adjust treatments, and provide support as new challenges come up.

During these follow-ups, the doctor will likely ask about your loved one's memory, mood, and behavior to see if anything has changed. They might check how well your loved one is managing daily activities like eating, dressing, or taking medications. Sometimes, the doctor may do physical exams or memory tests to see how things are progressing.

Expect to talk about any medications your loved one is taking and whether they are helping or causing side effects. The doctor might adjust doses or try new treatments depending on how things are going. If there are any concerns about safety at home, like falls or getting lost, the doctor might provide advice or suggest other professionals, like occupational therapists, to help.

It's really important to stay on top of any changes you notice with your loved one after a dementia diagnosis. Even small things, like changes in mood, memory, or behavior, can give the doctor an insight into how the condition is developing. So, don't hesitate to bring up anything new you've noticed, even if it seems minor.

Sharing this information proactively might allow the doctor to adjust treatments or suggest other strategies to manage the condition more effectively. If the medication doesn't seem to be working or is causing side effects, make sure that you mention that to your elderly's doctor. The doctor might then suggest alternatives or tweak the dosage to make things more comfortable for your loved one.

Also, make sure you ask any questions that are on your mind. The more you ask, the more you and the doctor might be able to work together for your elderly's betterment. Remember, you're not just following a treatment plan - you're part of a team with the doctor to make sure your loved one is as comfortable and supported as possible. The more you ask questions and share what's going on, the better the care may be.

Important Questions to Ask

After getting a dementia diagnosis of your loved one, you might be feeling anxious and unsure about what's next. It might be important to ask the doctor as many questions as possible. You can get an idea by looking at some questions put together by UCLA's Alzheimer's and Dementia Care Program.

Your loved one can ask these questions themselves if they're able to, and if they're not able to, you might ask in their place. Some of these questions are:

- What type of dementia do I have?

- What's the difference between Alzheimer's and dementia?

- What caused my dementia?

- What will happen as the disease gets worse?

- Besides memory loss, what other symptoms might I experience, and how quickly will things decline?

- Is there anything I can do to slow down this decline?

- What do you think about supplements and programs that say they can cure Alzheimer's?

- Where can I find more information about dementia?

- What support is available to help me through this?

- If I have a problem related to my dementia, who should I reach out to?

- How do I choose a family member or friend to be my caregiver?

- What goals should I set for myself now and down the road?

- As the disease progresses, will I experience pain?

- I worry about becoming dependent or being a burden. Will that happen?

- Should I share my diagnosis with others?

- Should I still spend time with people even if they notice changes in me?

- What are the chances my kids will get dementia? Can they do anything to prevent it?

Some additional questions you can ask the doctor might be:

- How can we change the treatment plan to help with new symptoms?

- What are the possible risks and benefits of changing medications?

- Are there any clinical trials for this type of dementia that we can consider?

It's okay to feel that there is too much on your plate because, honestly, that might be true. But what I want is for you to not forget to celebrate the wins, no matter how small they seem. Asking questions and staying open to different ideas might make a difference in your and your loved one's journey with dementia.

Chapter 8: Managing Behavioral Changes

I may have talked about this before here and there in this book, but as of now, I want to specifically address something or you could say a phenomenon that happens in dementia which is, in my opinion, so significant yet might get so easily disregarded, ignored, brushed off or not taken seriously. Given the title of this chapter, you may have guessed what I'm talking about. It's the behavioral changes that accompany this disease we know as dementia.

First off, if you're reading this, it is likely that you have a loved one who is undergoing something you might be confused about or you already know they have dementia. With the progress of this disease, it's common for people to show new and sometimes very different behaviors. Your loved one might start feeling more anxious or begin repeating questions, words, or actions over and over. This might catch you off guard, especially since these changes don't follow a set pattern - they come and go in surprising ways.

At first, you might have noticed this behavior and gotten a little upset on them on why they're repeating the same thing over and over again. Or, you might have said to them, "I just answered you. Why are you asking me the same thing again!?"

I want to highlight here that as the disease worsens, you may see them act in ways that seem unusual or out of character. They might become impulsive, saying or doing things that feel inappropriate or even a bit like how a child might behave. You might even notice them doing things that you just forbade them to do, or completely opposite of what they agreed on before. You might get surprised at this, even annoyed. And as a caregiver, this can be really hard, especially when you don't know what's going on or you're unfamiliar with something like this.

I want to share a story[27] here I read about a girl Lizzie who shared her father's story and wrote, *"My dad was a gentle giant in every sense. He was patient, kind and slow to anger. As father-daughter relationships go, ours couldn't have been stronger. Yes, he was my dad, but he was also one of my best friends."*

Lizzie then shared the early signs and diagnosis of her father and wrote, *"One of the earliest signs something wasn't right was with Dad's driving. He always did the long-haul driving when we'd go away, but he began to have trouble with the clutch and the gears. In 2017, we went on a family holiday to Canada. Dad was getting ready to drive us to the Airbnb, and he froze. He couldn't work out how to start the car, or process the directions we needed to go. We sat in that carpark for what felt like an eternity as he stared at the steering wheel. When we finally got to the accommodation, I broke down in tears. Dad cried too. We hugged and cried into each other's arms.*

Looking back, I knew something was wrong but I didn't think for a second that it was dementia."

Lizzie further shared that she had graduated from university and made the big move to London, where she was living with her best friends. She loved her new life in the city, and she was fully caught up in it.

---

[27] Dementia UK. (n.d.). *The greatest dad I could have ever asked for: Lizzie's story.* Dementia UK. https://www.dementiauk.org/information-and-support/stories/the-greatest-dad-i-could-have-ever-asked-for-lizzies-story/

But after a couple of years, things started to shift with her dad, and a quiet worry began settling in the back of her mind. She shared that she had started thinking more and more about how he was doing, even when she wasn't home. And every time she did visit, it became clear that things were getting harder for him. He'd begun staring off into space, not recognizing people the way he used to. Sometimes, he'd just stop in his tracks, looking confused and unsure of how to get home.

Lizzie further stated, *"He was diagnosed with young onset frontotemporal dementia in 2018, when he was 58 years old. I was 24. When I heard the news, I was at work. I remember thinking, I don't know how to feel right now. Yes, we finally had an answer to everything that had been going on for the past few years. But that answer was a condition with no cure. I didn't know how to handle that.*

I tried to go home as much as I could to support Mum with caring for Dad. A few years earlier, trips home would mean Dad spoiling me with fried breakfasts delivered to my bedroom and weekend bike rides, but now it was centered around how I could help care for my dad and provide support and respite for my mum..."

Lizzie shared that her dad's blank staring had gradually worsened. Taking him out in public became a source of stress - not just for him, but for the family as well. Being a tall man, people usually misread his distant look, assuming it was aggressive. Strangers would sometimes snap at him or, in some cases, even confront him as though he were a threat. It was heartbreaking to watch for her.

She further wrote, *"...I saw a practical opportunity to help the situation. I designed a t-shirt for Dad to wear – on the front it said, 'Sorry for staring, it's just my dementia'. The effect was almost*

125

immediate. Hostility was replaced with empathy and understanding...

In 2022, Dad was hospitalized for an infection. Following that, he was bed-bound in our family home. Prior to this, he had also become non-verbal. And while we found ways to find joy, it was a devastating time for all of us...

Dad died in May, 2024, in his own bed, with family at his side..."

I assume that after reading Lizzie's story, you might have felt a few or a lot of things relatable. You could have even felt the heartache that comes with dementia, both for the person living with it and for the loved ones who care for them. Like many others, Lizzie found that knowing the diagnosis brought her a sense of direction.

And so, it brings us back to what we were discussing about the symptoms when we don't know what's happening. Like Lizzie didn't understand what was going on with her dad on their trip to Canada in that parking lot, you might have gone through a similar situation too. But once you get to know what has happened to the brain i.e., the actual diagnosis, then you might start to research on it a bit and get to understand things. Knowing that the changes are part of the disease might make them a little easier to handle.

People with dementia usually lose the ability to express themselves before they lose the ability to understand what's happening around them. This means that their behavior often becomes their way of communicating. Along with other symptoms, dementia might also cause behaviors like wandering, agitation, anxiety, depression, and resistance to care.

These changes in behavior usually happen because dementia slowly affects parts of the brain that handle memory, decision-making, and emotions. As the disease progresses, people with dementia can get frustrated or anxious because they're losing abilities they used to have. They might forget people, places, or routines that they were once used to, which might make them feel lost and confused. Since they recurrently can't find the right words to share their feelings, they may repeat questions, act out, or seem withdrawn.

In simple terms, their behavior isn't done on purpose. It's a way of reacting to the changes in their brain. These behaviors aren't intentional - they come from the way dementia changes a person's view of the world. With the progress of this disease, the person with dementia starts to live in an altered reality, where things that they might have been once familiar with may now seem strange or confusing. When they forget names, places, or even routines, it can be deeply disturbing for them, and their behavior might reflect this.

I want you to think about a scenario in which your loved one suddenly doesn't recognize their own home. They might wander around, looking for a 'different' home because, in their altered reality, the rooms now feel strange. The point I want to make here is that this might not be intentional - it's their brain struggling to connect memories and surroundings. So, they might feel lost or anxious in a place they've lived for years.

Or, they might start asking the same question over and over, like "Where is my mom?" even if their mother passed away long ago. In their reality, they may genuinely feel like a child searching for comfort or safety. They might not realize the time that has passed. Their repeated questions might be a way of reaching out for comfort in a world that suddenly feels unpredictable or frightening to them.

Sometimes, they may do things they would have avoided before, like taking someone else's belongings or becoming frustrated during simple tasks. It's not a choice; rather, they're reacting to confusion and frustration because they can no longer process things the way they used to. By seeing these behaviors as responses to their altered reality, we can better understand what they're experiencing and respond with gentleness and patience.

If your loved one is acting out in a way that's hard to understand, try asking yourself, "What are they trying to tell me?" Are they feeling anxious, uncomfortable, or lonely? Maybe they're in pain but can't explain it in words. If you look at their behavior as a message, you might be able to figure out what they need and find a way or two to help or calm them.

Here, I want to share some relatable examples of common behavioral challenges in dementia, along with some tips on how you might be able to handle them:

1. <u>Forgetting and Repeating Questions</u>

When your loved one starts asking the same question repeatedly, like "What time is dinner?", it can be frustrating. You might answer them, only for them to ask again a few minutes later, and it may feel like doing a chore again and again. But this happens because memory loss makes it hard for them to remember the answer, even moments after you've said it. They might not be doing it to be difficult; they might truly not recall asking before.

Tips:

- Try to stay patient, even though I understand it can be very tough. Just to try to remind yourself that your loved one might not be doing this on purpose.

128

- Consider posting a note with answers to common questions, like "Dinner is at 6 p.m." It might give them some reassurance and ease their worry about forgetting.

- Gently redirect them to something they enjoy doing. This can sometimes help them relax and shift their focus.

2. Wandering

Your loved one might try to leave the house to go somewhere they remember, like an old workplace or a family member's home. This happens because they might feel like they're in a different time or place and don't realize they're already safe at home. Wandering usually signals a need for used to routines or a way to ease restlessness.

Tips:

- Try to make sure their environment is safe by installing locks out of sight or setting up security alerts.

- You can also try to engage them in an activity, like a short walk or a simple chore, to help them busy their mind.

- Try to stick to a daily routine. Familiarity might ease their anxiety and reduce wandering.

3. Resistance to Care

When it's time for a bath or a change of clothes, they might refuse, become frantic, or even push you away. They could be feeling vulnerable, confused, or embarrassed, especially if they don't fully understand the need for care. Everyday tasks might suddenly feel unaccustomed and even intimidating to them.

Tips:

- You can try to approach them calmly and gently explain each step. For instance, "Let's wash up mom, so we can feel fresh."

- You can also provide them choices to give them a sense of control, like asking if they'd prefer a bath now or in ten minutes.

- If they're strongly resistant, back off and try again later. Sometimes, a short break might make a difference.

4. <u>Aggression or Agitation</u>

You might see them suddenly become upset, raise their voice, or act out for no clear reason. As dementia affects their ability to express themselves, frustration or unmet needs (like hunger, pain, uncomfortableness or confusion) can result in outbursts. Something in the environment might also feel overwhelming to them.

Tips:

- Try to stay calm and avoid arguing with them. You can use a calming voice and gentle body language to help them feel safe.

- Try to look for triggers. Are they hungry? Are they tired? Are they comfortable? Are they in pain? Even small adjustments sometimes, like dimming the lights or making a change to the surrounding, might calm down your loved one.

- You can also try to redirect them to something that you think they might find comfort in.

In each of these situations, understand that their behavior is not deliberate. They might be responding to a world that feels strange to them. Staying calm and steering clear of confrontation is really important when handling these situations. People with dementia can pick up on our moods easily, so if we get frustrated or start arguing, it usually makes things worse. They might get even more confused or upset because they feel our tension, even if they can't fully understand the reason behind it.

Keeping calm, on the other hand, might help them feel safe. You can try to say things like, "I'm here for you, and it's okay." Sometimes, they just need that steady presence to calm their own worries. When we avoid arguing, we also avoid adding extra stress for everyone involved. Instead, we can focus on gently guiding them back to a more peaceful state, which usually makes things easier on both sides.

Strategies for Managing Behaviors

Caring for someone with dementia can look different for everyone. Sometimes you're right there, living with them, and other times you might be helping out from a distance. It might be a team effort, with family members or other caregivers pitching in to help. But no matter how close or far you are, being a caregiver might feel like a lot to handle.

When it comes to dementia, things don't always go the way we expect. It's not like there's a rule book for how to act or what to say, especially with memory loss. Even if something seems like it should make sense, it might not actually work in the moment. Here are some tips to keep in mind:

- **Validation:** I think that one of the most helpful ways to support someone with dementia is by using validation. This just means acknowledging what they're feeling, even if you don't fully understand it. When they're feeling confused, upset, or anxious, I think the most important thing is that they feel heard and cared for. For example, if they seem upset, you could say something like, "I can see that this is really bothering you," or "That must feel frustrating." You don't need to have all the answers. Just showing you understand that they're struggling can help them feel safer and more understood. Even if their concerns don't make sense to you, try not to dismiss them. Sometimes, just knowing you're listening and that you're there can make a big difference for you loved one.

- **Logic Doesn't Always Work:** If your loved one says or does something that feels a bit 'off,' it's only natural to want to explain things, hoping they'll understand and follow along. But with dementia, you need to remember that their mind doesn't work the same way as ours anymore. Instead of explaining too much, try using short, simple sentences about what's happening. It can keep things clear and help you both stay calm.

- **Reality Might Be Different for Them:** People with dementia may forget important things, even things as big as the passing of a loved one. Reminding them might only cause them to feel that sadness all over again. And when they say they want to 'go home,' telling them they're already home can lead to them getting frustrated. Instead, try gently shifting their attention. You could ask about the person or place they're talking about, so that they feel heard without adding stress.

- **Agreements Might Be Tricky:** Asking them to remember not to do something or to follow a rule often doesn't stick. They may mean to remember, but dementia makes it hard to follow through. Early on, a note might work, but later, making simple changes to their environment is more effective. For example, an automatic shut-off kettle can be used to avoid accidents, instead of just asking them to remember to turn it off.

- **Redirection:** When your loved one is stuck on something or starting to feel upset, gently steering their attention elsewhere can ease up the situation. You might say something like, "Let's go look at the flowers outside" or suggest another activity. This shift in focus might calm them and relieve any frustration they're feeling.

- **Simplification:** People with dementia can get overburdened with too many instructions or details. Breaking things down into small, clear steps might be the way to go. Instead of saying, "Let's get dressed, wash up, and then eat breakfast," try, "Let's start by putting on your shirt." Keeping things simple and focusing on one thing at a time might reduce confusion and make things feel more manageable.

- **Maintaining Routines:** Routines are very comforting for people with dementia. Having meals, baths, and other activities at the same time each day might create a sense of stability and reduce anxiety for your loved one. If you need to make changes to the routine, try to do it slowly to avoid too much confusion.

Focus on Communication

I understand that talking with someone who has dementia can be really tough, but with patience and kindness, it can be made a lot easier. When you speak clearly and gently, your loved one might feel understood and safe, even if they're feeling confused or struggling to remember things. The goal is to make them feel comfortable and valued.

Here are some simple ways to connect better and communicate with your loved one in a better manner:

- **Use Non-Verbal Cues:** Sometimes words might just not be enough. A smile, a gentle touch on the hand, or just nodding can go a long way. These non-verbal cues can show that you care and are listening, even if they're having a hard time following the conversation.

- **Keep Eye Contact:** Looking them in the eye shows you're really there with them. It might make them feel seen and understood. Plus, it makes the conversation feel more personal and focused, which is really important.

- **Speak Slowly and Gently:** Try to talk a bit slower than usual, and use simple words. It gives them time to think and respond without feeling rushed. It's okay to pause; sometimes, a little silence can actually make things easier to understand.

By using these little tips, you can make the conversation feel calmer and more connected. I understand that these tips might not always be easy to follow, but they might make a big difference for your loved one.

Part III:
Senior Care Options

Chapter 9: Aging Well at Home

I can understand how hard it can be to figure out the best care for your loved one. It might feel like there are so many options, and it can be tough to know what's right. You might be questioning yourself, *Can I care for Mom at home? Will I be able to do it myself alone? Would it be safe? Should I contact some care facility?* The idea of moving your loved one to a care facility itself might bring a ton of emotions, and apart from all this, your loved one might just want to stay at home themselves.

That's why many families choose in-home care. It lets your loved one stay in the place they know and love: their own home. You can imagine that they might find it comforting to be surrounded by their own people, their routines, and the memories they've built over the years.

Why Aging in Place Could Be a Good Choice?

Let's quickly have a look at why home care can be a great option for your loved one. It's simple, really - it might give them the support they need while keeping things comfortable. Here's the scoop:

- **They Stay Independent:** With home care, your loved one might get the help they need but can still do things their way. It can be hobbies, daily routines, or meeting friends; they might be able to keep their independence while getting the support that fits their life.

- **Great for Their Mind:** Being at home can be good for their mental health too. Surroundings that they are familiar with can help with memory and emotional welfare, which could make them feel more secure and happy.

- **It Saves Money:** Let's be honest, care homes can be pricey. Home care is usually more budget-friendly because you pay for just the time your loved one needs help. It can be considered a win-win: great care without breaking the bank.

- **Tailored Just for Them:** Home care can be completely personalized, meaning that your loved one gets care that matches their exclusive needs. Plus, they might get one-on-one attention from their caregiver.

- **You Might be Able to Stay Involved:** With home care, you're not limited by visiting hours. You or any other family member can drop by whenever it works for them and your loved one, which might help in keeping that connection and staying involved in their care.

- **Quicker Recovery:** Here's a fact: people tend to heal faster at home. Being in a known space helps recovery and lowers the risk of infections, which might mean fewer trips back to the hospital.

Why a Safe Home is So Important for Your Loved One?

Well, most seniors want to stay in their own homes and who can blame them? It's where they feel comfortable and independent. But as they age, especially if memory or behavior changes come into play, making their home a safe place becomes really important.

You might be thinking, *What kinds of safety issues could there be?* One big one is clutter. It's not unusual for seniors to resist decluttering or letting go of possessions. It could be sentimental for them, or they just don't see it as a problem. But too much stuff can make their home less safe, which could increase the chances of accidents.

So, how do you handle this? With patience and compassion. It might not be easy for them to part with things, and that's okay. Approach the conversation gently and focus on making changes together. Try to make them feel involved, not forced.

You might also wonder, *Is it really urgent to do this now?* Absolutely. A safe home doesn't just protect your loved one from accidents but it might also make caregiving less stressful for you. And also, it might give you a little peace of mind, knowing you're doing something to keep them healthy and happy at home. Remember, little positive changes now might make a big difference later.

Home Modifications for Your Loved One

More and more seniors are choosing to age in their own homes instead of moving to assisted living. But for this to work properly, they might need the right support and a safe and secure environment. With age, certain hazards can pop up in the home that might need to be carefully managed. Your elderly might be able to enjoy their independence safely and with confidence with the right preparation and care.

<u>Preventing Falls</u>

First things first, falls are a big risk for seniors, and we need to take steps to prevent them. In fact, falls are the leading cause of injury for people over 65. So, start with simple fixes like improving lighting, putting up handrails on stairs and porches, and keeping walkways clear of debris. Also, clean up spills right away and encourage your loved one to wear shoes that fit them well; for example, flat or low-heel shoes work best for balance.

Fire Safety

Did you know seniors are twice as likely to die in a fire compared to younger people? So, check smoke alarms regularly and change the batteries every year. Replace your smoke detectors every ten years. Make sure there's one on every floor, and avoid open flames, especially near oxygen. I would also recommend having flashlights with charged batteries instead of candles, which I think is a safer choice, too.

Try to Prevent Poisoning Hazards

Seniors, especially those dealing with dementia or confusion, are at risk of accidental poisoning, like mixing up medications or using expired ones. To help avoid this, keep medications in their original containers, throw away old meds, and make a medication schedule. You could also use a pill organizer to make it easier for them to take the right meds at the right time.

Medical Alert Systems

It can be considered a good option to have something like a medical alert system in place. These systems allow your loved one to call for help in an emergency, like if they fall or have health issues. There are systems that are monitored 24/7, or you can choose one that alerts family or friends when help is needed.

Make Your Home More Comfortable and Accessible

I think that anyone who loves their elderly would want to provide them with a space where they are comfortable as well as safe. For that, where do you start? Well, let's break it down by room to keep things simple.

Bathroom

In the bathroom, make sure the water heater is set to no more than 120°F. You don't want to risk a scalding accident. Grab bars in the shower or by the toilet are a must for balance, in my opinion, and rubber mats can be used to avoid slips. You can also make things easier by adding a raised toilet seat and a tub chair for more support. And don't forget to store medications and cleaning products out of reach - safety first!

Hallways and Stairs

For hallways and stairs, try to clear the pathways. Remove any throw rugs or clutter that could cause a trip. Installing sturdy handrails along stairs can make a big difference too. You also don't want any loose wires around, so make sure cords are tucked away safely.

Kitchen

In my opinion, the main point in this area of the house is simplicity. Go for appliances with easy-to-read controls, and make sure your kettle has an automatic shut-off to avoid boiling accidents. Store cleaning supplies away from food and use childproof locks if needed. It might also be a good idea to keep sharp items, like knives, in a safe, visible spot, like a rack, instead of a drawer.

Living Area

You might want to make sure there's nothing in the way that could cause a fall in the living area. Try to keep emergency numbers visible and easy to grab in case of a crisis. It could also be a good idea to declutter the space to make it easier to move around and process the surroundings. For fire safety, have fire extinguishers in main spots, like the kitchen and near bedrooms. Also, don't forget to check smoke and carbon monoxide detectors regularly.

Role of Lighting in Senior Home Safety

When you think about caring for your elderly loved one, lighting might not be the first thing that might come to mind, but it should be. The right lighting can greatly affect their mood, safety, and health. Have you ever thought about how light can influence their daily life beyond just seeing clearly?

Natural light can be considered one of the most beneficial sources. You can consider it as a natural mood booster, which helps to regulate their circadian rhythm and improve sleep. Exposure to sunlight triggers the production of serotonin, which can reduce anxiety and depression. Plus, natural light provides essential vitamin D and supports bone health and the immune system.

Now, let's talk about color temperature. It might sound like a small thing, but it can really influence how your loved one feels. Warm colors like yellow or orange tend to create a cozy, inviting atmosphere. On the other hand, cooler tones like blue can create a calming environment, which is particularly accommodating for those with vision issues or cognitive problems. Have you noticed how certain colors in a room can either energize or calm you down? I think that the right choice here might improve their comfort and even help them to sleep better.

Layered lighting is another part of this scenario, which is a mix of overhead, task, and accent lighting. This flexibility allows you to adjust the lighting to suit different activities, like reading, eating, or just relaxing.

Then there's smart lighting, which can be considered a modern solution to meet their unique needs. With features that mimic natural light and can be controlled remotely, you can have a lighting system that adjusts to their health needs throughout the day. Think about it for a moment. They could adjust the lighting with just a voice command, which obviously could be very convenient for some seniors.

Of course, glare-free lighting is important too. Glare can cause discomfort and uneasiness and even lead to accidents, especially for seniors with vision issues. Using lampshades or diffusers can soften the light and might make the environment more pleasant and reduce strain on their eyes.

Choosing The Right In-Home Care

I can understand that deciding to bring a paid caregiver into your home can be a big step for you. It can feel too much like you're admitting you can't do it all. But the thing is that it's not about giving up. You can think about it this way: you're trying to make sure your loved one stays safe, comfortable, and independent. You might wonder, *What does hiring a caregiver really mean? What do they even do?*

Basically, in-home care tries to keep individuals comfortable and independent in their own homes. Care plans are typically customized with a case manager to meet specific needs. But it just isn't limited to that since caregivers are supposed to bring emotional support, kindness, and connection to the table, which might make a big difference.

So, what exactly do caregivers do? Maybe you're thinking, *Is it just light housekeeping or more involved tasks?* Well, I would say that it depends. Caregivers assist with daily routines like meal prep, tidying up, sorting mail, or even grocery shopping.

They also handle personal care tasks like bathing, dressing, and mobility assistance. Some even offer overnight supervision or transportation to appointments. Their role can be as varied as the needs of the person they're caring for.

When you're hiring a caregiver, it's important to look for specific skills. Have you thought about what 'hard skills' really mean in this context? It's the basic medical knowledge that is a must - things like understanding medications or spotting symptoms. They should also know first aid and have the know-how to use medical devices like blood pressure monitors or wheelchairs. Equally important might be their ability to handle personal care and meal preparation tailored to the dietary needs of your elderly.

But technical skills are only half the story. Personality is also important and this is where the soft skills come into play that you should look for in the caregiver while hiring them. Things like empathy, communication, and emotional resilience can be considered some important traits here. Caregiving is deeply personal work, and a caregiver's ability to connect with your loved one can make a lot of difference in their mental health. Look for someone who listens patiently, adapts to changing needs, and stays calm under pressure. And don't forget about time management because juggling multiple tasks while staying attentive takes real skill.

You might be thinking, *How do I know if someone has all these qualities?* Start with a conversation. Ask about their experience, but also listen for warmth in how they talk about their work. You might want to trust your instincts here because finding someone who feels like the right fit can be just as important as their qualifications on paper.

Evaluating and Hiring a Caregiver

Choosing the right caregiver for your loved one might feel daunting, even scary. After all, stories about elder and child abuse remind us just how grave this decision can be. But don't let fear take over and try to do your best to find the right caregiver.

So, how do you find the right person? Even if a caregiver comes highly recommended, take time to thoroughly evaluate them. Let me share some tips:

- First, check their references. Ask multiple people about the caregiver's character and work ethic. How do they interact with the people they've cared for? Do they handle challenges well? Don't stop at one glowing review - dig deeper.

- Next, ask about a background check. You might question, *Is this really necessary?* Yes, it is. If the caregiver hesitates, that might be a red flag. While no check is foolproof, you can consider it as an important part of the screening process.

- Another tip is to run a quick search on the National Sex Offender Public Website (NSOPW). It pulls together information from registries across the U.S., so you can easily check by name or region. You might also look into their public social media or legal records for extra reassurance.

- Also, try to stay involved. Drop by unannounced once in a while to see how things are going. Are they providing the level of care you expect? These surprise visits might tell you a lot.

- Another tip is to educate yourself on the signs of elder abuse. Stay alert for unusual changes in mood, unexplained injuries, or sudden withdrawal.

Now that you have an idea about what to look for in a caregiver, the question coming to your mind could be, *Where do I actually find one?* Home care agencies can be considered an option that offers vetted caregivers and handles hiring and screening for you. Also, local colleges and nursing schools can connect you with trained graduates, usually through their placement programs. Online platforms, as well as job sites and community groups, make it easy to post jobs and review candidates. Lastly, personal recommendations from friends or family can provide leads and firsthand insights. Take your time to explore these options and try to find the best fit for your loved one's needs.

Interviewing the Caregiver

Once you have shortlisted some people, it's time for the meeting and interview them. Here, asking the appropriate questions to properly evaluate them can be considered important because I think through the questions, you'll be able to evaluate their skills, experience, and compatibility with your loved one. It might also be a good idea to include your elderly in the conversation to make sure they feel comfortable and their preferences are considered. Here are some questions you can ask:

- Can you share your experience providing care for elderly patients?

- How would you handle a situation if a person refuses to take their medication?

- Tell me about a time you dealt with a medical emergency, and can you tell me what happened?

- How do you make sure about dignity and privacy during personal care tasks?

- What's your approach to handling emotional challenges, especially with seriously ill or end-of-life clients?

- How do you manage stress, particularly with difficult patients?

- Have you worked with clients who have dementia or mobility issues? How do you approach their care?

- How would you respond if a client falls or gets injured?

- What experience do you have caring for someone with depression?

- How do you balance senior independence with safety?

- How would you handle a disagreement with someone under your care?

- Can you recall a time when you had to share difficult news with a family member? How did you do it?

- Are you familiar with preparing meals for people with diabetes?

- Have you dealt with a client who was abusive or difficult? How did you handle it?

- What would you do if a client confided in you something that should be shared with their family or healthcare team?

Building a Relationship with Your Elderly Loved One's Caregiver

Once you have hired a caregiver, you might want to build a nice relationship with them. This might take some time, trust, and clear communication. It can feel a little tricky at first, especially since your loved one might hesitate to ask for help and might want to stay independent. But as the caregiver shows kindness, respect, and reliability, trust might naturally grow. Make sure to talk openly about what works, what doesn't, and any concerns because in my opinion, clear-cut and open communication might help a lot in avoiding confusion and building understanding. You have to remember that being patient is important, especially while everyone gets used to each other. Try to spend some quality time together, like going for walks or sharing small activities to create a warm and supportive connection.

Elderly Care Using Technology

Home healthcare has come a long way from being a luxury for the privileged to becoming a widely accessible solution due to the help of modern technology. Today, digital tools have helped in making healthcare more inclusive and they benefit not just seniors but also people with special needs, those recovering from medical setbacks, and people managing chronic conditions. With innovations like online consultations and digital medical records, patients can now receive efficient care from the comfort of their homes.

Home Monitoring Systems

In-home monitoring systems are becoming a way to support the health and safety of older people who live on their own. These systems can keep an eye on your loved one at home or even when they're out and about. These systems work in two ways: **active** and **passive.** Active systems need some action, like pressing a button to call for help. Passive systems, on the other hand, do the job automatically - no need for your loved one to do anything, which can be very helpful if they fall or are unable to respond.

Here, I want you to think about your loved one's particular needs. For health concerns, wearable devices might be a good choice, as they can send real-time health data straight to doctors. If falls are a worry, a simple call button with a two-way speaker could be a good option. Active seniors who are usually on the move might prefer a device with GPS, which could provide you with a bit of peace of mind while they're out.

If your loved one is healthy but maybe feeling isolated, wellness trackers that monitor sleep, activity, or medication schedules could be worth considering. For those with dementia, a system with cameras or motion sensors might give you a little more reassurance. Many systems even connect to free apps, so you can stay in the loop if medications are skipped or if they're moving around late at night.

In my opinion, the best systems are simple and easy to use. There are features like a water-resistant wearable, fall detection, and a two-way speaker, which I think can be particularly helpful. When choosing one, ask yourself: Does it have a good range? Can it be worn comfortably as a wristband or necklace? How long does the battery last? And if you want more coverage, do you need one with cameras? Basically, I would say just consider what might be the most useful considering your elderly's needs.

Telehealth and Remote Healthcare Services

Telehealth can be said to be changing the game when it comes to caring for your elderly loved ones. Have you noticed how much easier life feels when healthcare comes to us rather than the other way around? With telehealth, your elderly can consult doctors, manage medications, and monitor their health without leaving the comfort of home. I think it's a smart, cost-effective way to make healthcare more accessible, especially if mobility or transportation is an issue.

This shift is empowering for seniors, too. They get to take an active role in their health through virtual consultations or tools that track things like blood pressure or blood sugar. And because providers can adjust treatment plans in real-time, telehealth brings a more personalized, higher-quality care experience.

One of the best parts, I think, is the convenience. Your loved one can access care anytime with just a phone or computer. Moreover, medication management also gets a boost. With telehealth tools, healthcare providers can keep track of schedules and dosages and avoid dangerous medication errors.

That said, telehealth isn't perfect. Some seniors might find smartphones or computers tricky, especially if they have vision, hearing, or cognitive problems. The good news is that there are resources like screen readers or voice-to-text programs that have become more common to help bridge the gap.

I think that all of this ties into something very important: the importance of home. For many seniors, home isn't just a building but a space filled with their memories and comfort. Aging in place might let them stay connected to what they know and love.

Chapter 10: Making the Move to Assisted Living

By now, you probably understand how important it is for your elderly loved one to hold on to their independence. It might be one of the biggest fears many seniors have, and it's easy to see why – they might have spent their whole lives being self-reliant. Most seniors want to stay in their own homes, but we realize that many elderly people need help with daily activities. So, how can they get the support they need without giving up their independence? That's where assisted living comes in.

You might be wondering, *What exactly is assisted living?* Well, I would say it might be considered somewhat of a middle ground. It's not quite the independence of living on your own, but it might be far from the hospital-like environment of a nursing home. Assisted living communities provide personalized care in a residential setting for older adults who need some help but still want to maintain their autonomy. The level of support might be personalized to each resident, with a focus on promoting a healthy and socially active lifestyle.

These communities are designed to feel like home while offering the assistance seniors need. It could include help with medication, meals, or other daily tasks; the goal is to strike a balance - provide care while encouraging as much independence as possible.

What Kind of Services Do They Provide?

When someone moves into an assisted living community, they typically undergo an assessment to create a customized plan based on their unique needs to make sure their care feels personal and meets them where they are.

Now, one of the questions that hangs during these types of conversations is about the costs. Assisted living usually involves a base monthly rent for the living space, with extra fees for additional services like help with daily activities or specialized care. The basic rent usually includes essentials like a private living space (which ranges from cozy studios to larger apartments), maintenance, an emergency alert system, daily meals, housekeeping, laundry, scheduled transportation, and activities like classes or outings to keep residents active and engaged.

For the elderly who might be in need of more support, extra services can be added for an additional fee. These might include help with eating, bathing, toileting, or medication management, access to on-site pharmacies or doctors, grooming services like haircuts, and even faster WiFi for tech-savvy seniors.

The good thing about assisted living is its flexibility, I would say, as residents can choose the level of support they need while still enjoying an independent lifestyle.

The Move to Assisted Living Might Be a Big Decision

When you finally sit down and think about deciding to move your loved one to an assisted living facility, I can somewhat understand how you might feel. It is a big step, and it's natural to have mixed feelings about it. If your loved one is having difficulty with everyday tasks like bathing, dressing, or cooking, assisted living might be a good solution.

You might wonder, *is assisted living the right fit?* Typically, residents in these communities can still live mostly on their own but need some help with daily activities. They should have a level of mobility and not require constant medical supervision.

This transition usually comes at the time when aging at home becomes too difficult. Assisted living aims to provide a safe, supportive environment where your loved one can stay active, social, and well cared for.

What Are the Types of Assisted Living Communities?

Small Residential Homes

When staying at home gets too hard for your elderly loved one, small residential homes can be a good option. These homes feel more like a family setting, far from the big, formal vibe of traditional facilities. They are known as residential care homes or adult family homes and are usually located in regular neighborhoods and provide personal care in a warm and close-knit environment.

You might ask, *what's special about small residential homes?* Unlike bigger places, these homes typically take care of ten or fewer residents, which might create a friendly and peaceful space that might be nice for your senior if they enjoy quiet surroundings or close connections. They help with everyday tasks like grooming, using the bathroom, and getting around while letting seniors keep as much independence as possible.

Residents might get to enjoy home-cooked meals, shared living areas, and a relaxed, homely feel. Services might include help with daily activities, laundry, cleaning, and managing medications. While these homes don't usually provide medical care, they might have staff available 24/7 for emergencies. Though smaller in size, these homes might plan group outings, simple activities, and ways for seniors to stay socially active.

The Good and The Bad of Small Residential Homes

Small residential homes have many advantages that can make them a great choice for your loved one. Their smaller size means more one-on-one attention, which might be due to a better staff-to-resident ratio. The convenient, home-like setting might provide a sense of comfort and familiarity, which might make it easier for your loved one to settle in. Moreover, management is usually approachable and flexible, which might make communication between staff, residents, and families much smoother.

Furthermore, these homes might allow for a more personalized experience. For example, residents might enjoy meals that suit their tastes or add personal touches to their space. With fewer people, the risk of illnesses spreading, like the flu or COVID, might be lower, and there's also a reduced chance of falls or other health issues.

However, small residential homes come with their challenges. They're in high demand, so finding an available spot may involve a waitlist. Compared to larger facilities, they may have fewer amenities, like gyms or pools, which could be important to some elderly people.

Also, small homes usually charge more, which can strain a budget. They may also be limited in their ability to provide advanced care if your loved one's needs change over time, such as with progressing dementia. Financial stability can be a concern, too, as some smaller homes may close within a decade of opening. Also, for the elderly who enjoy socializing, the smaller group size might feel limiting compared to larger communities.

Remember that each home might be a little different, so it's important to look for one that matches your loved one's needs and personality. For seniors who want a quieter life with personal attention and a comfortable space, small residential homes can be a nice choice.

Larger Assisted Living Facilities

Larger assisted living facilities can be a good choice if your elderly loved one values variety and resources. These communities typically provide more services, like gyms, pools, etc. If your loved one enjoys staying active, meeting new people, or participating in group activities, they might like this environment. On the other hand, some might find structured schedules less accommodating, especially if they have specific routines or habits they enjoy.

One thing to keep in mind is that larger facilities every so often have the ability to adapt to changing needs. For example, they usually provide multiple levels of care. If dementia or other health problems become a concern, these communities usually have dedicated staff and resources to provide specialized care. In my opinion, this continuity can be a huge relief.

You may also be thinking about the level of attention your loved one would get. It's true that larger facilities can feel a bit less personal compared to smaller homes. While they strive to provide quality care, the size can make one-on-one interactions less frequent. Still, they usually have highly skilled staff and administrators who are experienced in providing for a wide range of needs. If you're worried about this, I'd recommend asking about staff-to-resident ratios during your visits and observing how engaged the staff are with residents.

Safety is another consideration. Larger communities are usually well-equipped to handle emergencies and can dedicate entire wings for residents with contagious illnesses, like during the COVID-19 pandemic. However, a higher number of people can increase the risk of transmission. If this is a concern for you, it's worth discussing their infection control protocols in detail.

When you're choosing a facility, think about your loved one's personality and preferences. Are they someone who blooms in social settings with lots of activities? Or do they prefer quiet, personal time? For introverts, a smaller residence might feel cozier and more comfortable. But for extroverts, a larger community might provide the atmosphere they need to feel at home.

The Good and the Not-So-Good of Large Assisted Living Facilities

When you're considering a larger assisted living facility, there might be several factors to weigh. On the bright side, these communities usually have more availability, which can make finding a room much easier compared to smaller, more exclusive options. Financial stability is another significant plus since many larger facilities are backed by corporations. If you're looking for a range of care options, larger residences typically have you covered, as they might provide everything from assisted living to specialized memory care with on-staff nurses.

Amenities are another thing. Larger communities frequently feature perks like gyms, etc. If your loved one is social and enjoys meeting new people, they'll likely appreciate the many opportunities for interaction in these full-of-go communities. And surprisingly, larger facilities can be considered more cost-effective than smaller ones, which can be a relief if you're balancing care needs with a budget.

That said, there are trade-offs. You might find that larger facilities lack the cozy, homely feel of smaller residences, sometimes resembling a hospital or hotel instead. Staff in these settings can be more focused on routines than individual needs, which might affect the level of personalized care. Also, with more residents to look after, one-on-one attention can be harder to come by.

Management in larger facilities, especially those run by corporations, may also feel less accessible. If you have concerns or need to discuss your loved one's care, you might find it more difficult to connect with decision-makers.

Another thing to consider is health and safety. Larger communities can face greater challenges in containing illnesses like the flu or COVID simply because of the number of people living and working there. Additionally, statistics suggest a higher incidence of falls in larger facilities, which is something to keep in mind if mobility or balance is already a concern.

Ultimately, you would need to think about finding the right fit. Spend time visiting a few facilities, ask questions, and imagine your loved one there. Maybe you'll realize you've found the right place when it feels like it could be their new home and not just a facility.

Specialized Assisted Living Options

To talk about specialized assisted living options, let's focus on Alzheimer's care as an example to see how this type of facility works. I would like you to consider a scenario. For example, your elderly loved one is in a place where the staff is trained as well as deeply compassionate. Usually, the staff in these facilities seem to receive expert guidance and are chosen for their empathy and warmth, which might be considered an important factor when dealing with an Alzheimer's patient. They try to care for the residents as well as connect with them.

Activities in these facilities are usually carefully planned to engage the mind, with games and programs designed to create new memories or slow mental decline. I think you'd be surprised by how effective these can be, especially with the use of innovative learning tools.

And then there's the peace of mind that comes with round-the-clock care. Knowing that someone is always there to assist and comfort your loved one might lift a huge weight off your shoulders. You might be wondering, "Can they really care for my loved one as I would?" Many families find that these caregivers provide a level of attention that feels like an extension of their own love and devotion.

I can understand that caring for someone with Alzheimer's is no small task, and it can be just too much. That's why these specialized living options might be helpful.

What Should I Look for in an Assisted Living Community?

Choosing the right assisted living facility for your elderly loved one can feel like a big task, but breaking it down might make it easier. Start by asking questions and planning visits to see the facilities in person. If you can, visit at different times of the day or even drop in unannounced, as it might give you a clearer picture of daily life there. If visiting isn't an option, many places offer live virtual tours, which might still be helpful.

When you tour, pay attention to how the staff interacts with residents. Do they seem kind, patient, and respectful? You might ask here, "Will they treat my loved one like family?" In my opinion, you can usually tell by how they talk to and care for the residents. Don't be shy about asking about their training and background.

Next, take a look at the rooms. Are there different sizes or layouts? Would your loved one prefer a private room, or are they okay with sharing? It's worth thinking about whether the space feels welcoming, like somewhere they'd enjoy living.

Cleanliness matters too. Is the facility tidy and well-kept? Are the residents clean and well-groomed? I think these little details can tell you a lot about the level of care being provided.

Dining is another big piece. If you can, try a meal during your tour. You might even chat with residents to hear what they think about the food and daily life. Some facilities have resident ambassadors who can share their experiences, which can be a nice way to get feedback.

Also, safety should be a top priority. Are hallways and common areas free of clutter? Do they have security measures like medical alert systems?

Finally, consider the cost and future care. Make sure you understand how pricing works and if the facility can adapt to your loved one's needs if their health changes. You might have in mind, "What happens if they need more care down the road?" So, ask them about this as well.

A Glimpse into Assisted Living

Staying Active and Engaged

Your elderly loved one might stay active and engaged in an assistive living facility as there are usually scheduled events like weekly activities to keep residents busy and excited. They might also get to do exercises like stretching or group walks. I think group activities like these might help them to stay social and make new friends. They might also like it a lot if they're of an extrovert nature.

Moreover, your loved one might be able to keep their mind sharp with book clubs or guest speakers. Assisted living usually makes it easy to try something new or dive into old hobbies.

I would like to highlight here that moving to assisted living doesn't mean losing touch with family. In fact, family members are usually welcome to join social events or share a meal.

Nutrition and Dining

Meals are a big deal in assisted living. They try to focus on making meals that are both delicious and healthy. Your loved one might be sitting down to grilled salmon or spaghetti with garlic bread, chatting with others over dessert. Doesn't that sound nice?

The staff plans meals to suit different tastes and dietary needs. Residents usually get to choose their meals. Moreover, I think meals bring people together. Eating with others might help your elderly loved one feel less lonely and more at home.

If you asked for a menu of an assisted living facility, you might get to see something like this:

Breakfast

- Eggs, toast, and bacon
- Yogurt with berries
- Oatmeal or whole-grain cereals
- Coffee, orange juice, or milk

Lunch

- Beef Stroganoff
- Grilled cheese and tomato soup
- Fresh salads and light desserts

Dinner

- Grilled salmon or spaghetti
- Appetizers like soup or rolls
- Desserts like cake, ice cream, or sugar-free pudding

Preserving Dignity

You or your loved one might worry about maintaining independence when considering an assisted living option. Well, it's a common concern, but the goal of these communities is to support the elderly people while also helping them maintain their dignity and sense of control.

Why Does the Transition Feel Hard?

- Your loved one might feel like they're giving up control, which might affect their confidence.

- A new living space can feel uncomfortable and even unsettling at first.

- Your loved one might feel embarrassed about needing help with personal care, like dressing or bathing.

- Health problems or mobility issues might make it harder for them to join social activities, which might lead to loneliness.

How Should These Communities Promote Independence and Respect?

- Even small things, like choosing their clothes or grooming themselves, can help your loved one feel like an independent person.

- Bringing something personal into their room can make it feel more like home. You might think, "Will this really help?" In my experience, it might make a difference.

- I think seniors should have the freedom to make decisions about their daily routines, if they're capable of it. Respect from the staff might go a long way in preserving their dignity.

- Tools like emergency response systems or medication reminders might help your senior stay independent while having the safety net they need.

I think the bottom line here is that living in assisted living doesn't have to mean taking over but rather balancing support and independence.

Chapter 11: When Medical Needs Increase

When the medical needs of your loved one increase, it can become harder to manage and take care of them at home. Your loved one may require more frequent assistance, specialized care, or round-the-clock supervision. This is when exploring options like nursing homes or long-term care facilities might come into play.

You might wonder if a nursing home is the right option for your loved one. In my opinion, nursing homes can be considered a choice when exceptional care is needed. They're designed for both short-term recovery and long-term stays, which might be an option for seniors who require 24-hour medical attention or help with daily tasks like bathing or moving around.

If your elderly parent or loved one is dealing with a chronic illness, severe physical or cognitive problems, or complex medical needs that can't be managed at home, a nursing home might be an option. It's not an easy decision, but sometimes, it might be the way to make sure they receive the care and support they need.

You might hear terms like 'skilled nursing facility' and 'nursing home' and wonder if they mean the same thing. They often do! These facilities usually provide skilled nursing care along with rehabilitation and personal care. For example, skilled nursing could include wound care, managing insulin pumps, or care supervised by a registered nurse. If your loved one needs rehabilitation after an injury or illness, nursing homes usually provide physical therapy, occupational therapy, and even speech therapy to help them regain their independence.

Skilled Nursing Care

Your loved one might dream of aging comfortably at home - and who wouldn't? It's a thought I think most aged people would have. But as time passes, the needs of the elderly might increase in such a way that they might require special care.

So, what exactly is skilled nursing care? In simple terms, it's considered to be the medical care that can only be provided or supervised by licensed healthcare professionals like nurses, therapists, or even dieticians. It can happen in different places, like through home health agencies, assisted living communities with nurses, or skilled nursing facilities where 24/7 care is available.

You might be thinking, "Who provides this care?" A whole team of professionals can step in - Registered Nurses (RNs), Licensed Practical Nurses (LPNs), Certified Nursing Assistants (CNAs), and even physical or speech therapists. Their job is to provide care that exceeds what family members or outpatient services can manage but does not necessitate a hospital stay.

Skilled nursing care can also include things like IV treatments, wound care, pain management, or even help with medical equipment. Does your loved one need diabetes management, occupational therapy, or recovery care after surgery? These are all examples of where skilled nursing might make a big difference. It's usually the bridge between hospital care and returning to everyday life.

What's the Difference Between Assisted Living and Nursing Homes?

To answer this question, let's first recap what assisted living looks like. You can think of it as a middle ground between fully independent living and more intensive care. In these communities, your loved one can enjoy their independence but might still get help with things like meal preparation, medication reminders, or housekeeping. Assisted living is designed for seniors who need a little support while still maintaining a sense of autonomy.

Now, nursing homes are a step up in terms of care. They cater to people with more complex medical needs and provide 24/7 skilled nursing care. If your loved one requires constant medical attention or substantial help with daily tasks like bathing and mobility, a nursing home might be the right choice.

Let's have a closer look at the differences between them both to get a better idea.

- ## How Much Care Do They Really Need?

I think the biggest difference is the level of care. Nursing homes are equipped to handle more complex medical needs with 24/7 staffing, including registered nurses. This makes them ideal for seniors needing constant medical attention. On the other hand, assisted living focuses on helping residents with daily tasks like dressing or meal preparation while encouraging independence.

(And just to clarify, by saying "level of care," I mean to refer to the type of assistance provided, not the quality.)

- ## What Does the Place Feel Like?

Nursing homes have a clinical setup designed for medical care and safety, particularly for those prone to falls or wandering. While they might aim to be comfortable, the focus is on functionality. On the other hand, assisted living feels more like home. Residents might have private rooms or suites, and the atmosphere is usually more social and open.

- ## What About Personal Space?

In nursing homes, shared rooms are common, which might create a more communal vibe. Assisted living facilities typically provide private apartments or studios and give seniors their own space while still being part of a community. These communities emphasize recreation, with larger shared spaces for activities and gatherings.

- ## How Much Does It Cost?

Assisted living is generally more affordable than nursing homes, as the care provided is less intensive. Nursing homes, with their day-and-night medical care, can cost about twice as much. Don't let the numbers overwhelm you, though. However, many families are surprised to find assisted living more budget-friendly than expected after exploring their options.

- ## How Long Do People Stay?

The average stay differs between the two. Residents in assisted living usually stay one to two years, while nursing home stays average around 2.25 years. I think it's important to consider these timeframes when planning for the care needs of your elderly loved one.

- ## How Independent Can They Be?

Assisted living promotes more independence. Residents can come and go, drive themselves, and enjoy private living spaces. Nursing homes, however, have a more structured and supervised environment. Residents typically don't leave the facility without assistance or approval, as their care needs are greater.

So, Which Option Is Better?

This is where it might get tricky. I think the 'better' option depends on your loved one's needs. Assisted living might work well for those who value their independence but need a little help here and there. Nursing homes, on the other hand, might be better suited for people with higher healthcare needs or chronic conditions that might require continuous care.

Ultimately, the choice comes down to your loved one's specific situation. Take time to assess their medical needs, personal preferences, and what environment would make them feel most comfortable and supported.

Moving to a Nursing Home

When your elderly loved one is moving to a nursing home, you might get busy with packing boxes and gathering things that they might need. But I think that would not be the only thing swirling in your mind. You might have different kinds of emotions and thoughts, like how they would adjust, how the transition would be, if this was the right decision or not, etc. There might be emotional and practical aspects involved in this life-changing step. Let's walk through this together and explore how you can try to make this transition smoother for everyone involved.

- **What If They Feel Nervous?**

    It's natural to feel anxious about the unknown. You might wonder if your loved one will adjust or if they'll feel like they're losing independence. Take a deep breath - remind yourself (and them) that this move is about taking care of them better.

- **Saying Goodbye to the Familiar**

    Leaving a beloved home can feel like leaving a part of their identity behind. They may grieve the memories and comfort of their old space. Help them bring a piece of 'home' with them, like favorite blankets or beloved keepsakes, so that they make their new room feel warm and familiar.

- **Adjusting to the New Place**

    Structured routines in a nursing home can feel restrictive at first. Meal schedules, group activities, and caregiver interactions might take some getting used to. Encourage them to see it as a chance to embrace new things and create new habits.

- **Dealing with Family Guilt**

    Let's be real - making this decision can tug at your heartstrings. It's natural to feel guilty or second-guess if you're doing the right thing. But always keep in mind their care requirements and if you would be able to fulfill those needs at home. Ask yourself and then try to make the right decision that is best for your loved one.

- **Building New Connections**

    Meeting new people in a new environment might not be easy, especially for someone who's used to being independent.

Ask your loved one to join activities or simply share a meal with others. These small steps might lead to friendships and a sense of belonging.

The emotional side is only half the story. The practical details might require just as much care and attention. Let's have a look at how you might be able to approach these practical aspects.

- **Count the Costs**

When making the move, try to understand the financial requirements of nursing home care. Take the time to create a plan to manage long-term care expenses. With a clear budget in place, you might feel more prepared to handle the costs.

- **Declutter with Care**

Downsizing doesn't have to be daunting. Work together to decide what to keep, donate, or discard, and focus on items that bring comfort and practicality to their new space. Try to transform the decluttering process into an opportunity to share stories and create a fresh start in their new home.

- **Get Healthcare in Check**

Before the move, I would recommend you to have a thorough look at the medical care of your elderly. Try to make sure medical records are transferred, prescriptions are updated, and any ongoing treatments are accounted for.

- **Understand the Rules of the Road**

Every nursing home has its own policies and procedures, from visitation hours to how decisions are made. Get yourself acquainted with these guidelines early on so there are no surprises later. When you are informed, it might make communication and collaboration with the facility staff a little smoother.

- **<u>Keep the Lines Open</u>**

   Moving to a nursing home is a team effort. Try to maintain open, ongoing dialogue between family members, your loved one, and the facility's staff. Regular updates and clear communication might prevent misunderstandings.

- **<u>Plan the Big Day</u>**

   A well-organized move can make a huge difference. Create a timeline, make a checklist, and decide whether to hire professionals or take a hands-on approach. Packing your elderly's belongings, setting up their new room, etc., should be part of thoughtful planning to try to make sure the move feels smooth and stress-free.

Getting Used to a New Place

How can I make this transition easier?

Do you have this question in mind? Well, if yes, then I would guess that creating a supportive environment and finding ways to make the new setting feel comfortable and welcoming might be the thing you want for your loved one. So, let's explore some steps to go through this change.

As we mentioned earlier, emotions play a big role in this process. In my opinion, it's important to acknowledge the wide range of feelings both you and your loved one may experience – it can be sadness, anxiety, or even relief. You can consider these emotions normal. Give yourself and your loved one the grace and time to adjust. Talking to friends, family, or even a counselor can help you and your loved one process these feelings. Some nursing homes even offer support groups where residents and families can share their journeys.

Another important step, in my point of view, is to get familiar with the environment. Take time to explore the nursing home together - walk through common areas, check out the dining space, and peek into the recreational rooms. Knowing the layout might help to reduce anxiety and help the place feel less overwhelming. If you haven't had the chance to meet the staff or other residents, try to have a friendly conversation with them.

Also, personalizing your loved one's living style might be helpful. I think maintaining personal routines, like morning coffees or evening walks, can also bring comfort. What items or routines could help your loved one feel more grounded? That's the question you might want to ask yourself.

Also, after your loved one has made the move, you can encourage them to participate in nursing home activities. It can be an exercise class, a book club, etc., which can be an opportunity for them to meet others and stay engaged.

Skilled Nursing Facilities

Skilled Nursing Facilities (SNFs) might be considered a big part of caring for people with serious medical needs. You might be wondering, "What makes an SNF different from other care options?" I would say it's related to the specialized care they provide. What really sets SNFs apart is the team of skilled nurses, therapists, and healthcare experts. They help with things like physical therapy, wound care, or managing medications. If your elderly loved one is recovering from surgery or dealing with a chronic illness, an SNF might provide the structured care they need to feel safe and supported.

I think SNFs might also be good for people who need ongoing help. They do provide medical care but also try to create a place where residents can heal, stay active, and live as comfortably as possible.

In my experience, knowing what SNFs offer can make it easier to decide if they're the right choice.

Across-the-board Health and Rehabilitative Care

Skilled Nursing Facilities provide a wide range of medical services to support people with complex health needs. SNFs are designed to give 24/7 care, including help with medications, wound care, and monitoring vital signs. If your loved one needs constant medical attention, having licensed professionals on-site might make a difference.

One of the most important roles of SNFs is rehabilitation. They offer physical, occupational, and speech therapy to help residents recover from surgeries, illnesses, or injuries. These programs are usually personalized to fit each person's needs and goals. This individualized care might be important to help people rebuild their strength and regain independence.

SNFs take a team approach to care, involving doctors, nurses, therapists, social workers, and dietitians. This means they don't just focus on medical issues but also try to support emotional and social comfort.

For those recovering from hospitalization or surgery, SNFs might provide an important step toward independence. Rehabilitation focuses on improving mobility, strength, and everyday skills so residents can feel confident and capable again.

Professional Care Teams Might Be Important

Professional care teams can be considered the backbone of quality healthcare in settings like hospitals, clinics, nursing homes, and even home care. *But what makes these teams so important?* In my opinion, it's their ability to combine different skills and perspectives to provide the best care possible.

Care teams are made up of experts like doctors, nurses, therapists, social workers, and other specialists. Each brings their own knowledge to address different aspects of a patient's care. For example, while a physician might focus on diagnosis, a therapist can help with recovery and mobility.

These teams don't just look at the physical conditions but also consider emotional, social, and psychological well-being. In my opinion, this whole-person care might make a big difference in recovery and quality of life. Wouldn't it feel reassuring to know that your loved one's overall health is the priority?

Coordination and communication are also important. Professional care teams might work together to make sure everyone is on the same page about a patient's care plan. This might reduce errors, avoid repeated tests, and help things run smoothly. Have you ever experienced the frustration of uncoordinated care? Teams like this are designed to prevent that.

I also think it's important how much these teams value patient-centered care. They involve the patient in decisions and try to consider their preferences and goals.

Another advantage of professional care teams might be how quickly these teams can assess and adapt to a patient's needs. Regular discussions help them adjust care strategies as situations change. This flexibility might be a game-changer for someone dealing with a chronic illness or recovering from an injury.

I also think that working in a team encourages learning. Members share knowledge, stay updated on the latest treatments, etc. In my opinion, this constant improvement might benefit everyone.

Quality of Care

Good care in healthcare facilities is so important because it affects how well patients recover and how happy they are with the care they receive. Skilled Nursing Facilities provide nursing care, rehabilitation, and medical help as needed.

Each resident should have a care plan that is just for them. This plan looks at their medical needs, feelings, and social life. It should be checked and updated regularly to keep up with any changes.

I think a big part of good care depends on having enough staff who are well-trained. Staff members need regular training to keep improving how they care for people. Having enough workers might also be important to making sure every resident gets the attention they need.

Nutrition matters, too. SNFs need to serve healthy meals that meet residents' dietary needs and personal tastes. Nutritious food and proper hydration are important for staying strong.

Then again, communication might be just as important. Staff need to listen to residents and families and respect their rights, privacy, and dignity. When everyone talks openly and works together, it might make solving problems and meeting needs much easier.

How Can Inspection Reports Help You Choose a Nursing Home?

Inspection reports are documents created after a healthcare facility is inspected by government agencies or accrediting organizations. These reports check if the facility is following all rules and providing proper care.

In Skilled Nursing Facilities, inspection reports are a big deal. They look at important areas like how residents are cared for, safety measures, staff levels, and the overall environment. If a facility isn't meeting certain standards, the report might point out the problem and explain what needs to be fixed.

These reports usually include information about things like pain management, how often residents fall, and how satisfied residents are. Many of these reports are public and available online, which might be a big help for you if you're trying to choose the best place for your loved one.

You can consider inspection reports important to make sure SNFs provide high-quality care. Regular checks, open reporting, and fixing problems quickly help keep standards high and residents safe. For you, as the caregiver, these reports might be a great tool to compare facilities and make confident decisions.

To wrap it up, nursing homes, assisted living, and skilled nursing facilities all provide different types of care. You might need to understand what each one offers to find the best fit for your loved one's needs. I think choosing the option that feels right for their comfort and general health is important.

Part IV:
Thriving in Later Life

Chapter 12: Staying Active, Staying Independent

When it comes to supporting seniors, I think one of the biggest things that can make a difference is helping them stay independent. You might have noticed that as they get older, certain things, like moving around the house or even cooking meals, can become harder. But little changes might make it easier for them to keep living on their own.

Why Is Being Independent So Important for Your Loved One?

Let's take a moment to talk about why independence matters so much for seniors.

Losing independence can be tough for anyone, but it might be especially hard for seniors who've spent their whole lives making their own decisions, like raising families, building careers, and just being themselves. Aging can throw in some issues like mobility problems, isolation, or even financial worries. These things can make them feel like they're losing control over their lives.

And while we can't take away all the challenges of getting older, we can try to focus on how important independence is to their well-being. I think that keeping that sense of freedom and choice really matters - not just emotionally, but physically, too.

Helping Them Stay Themselves

You might have noticed that when your loved one feels in control, they seem more like themselves, right? That's because independence might make them able to express who they are. If they start to lose that, it might make them feel sad, angry, or even act out in ways that might surprise you.

One way to help might be to encourage them to keep their space personal. Let them decorate it with items that mean a lot to them. Maybe they have a favorite chair, a special quilt, etc.; you can ask them to keep those.

Another small but powerful way to help might be to give them choices. Simple things, like deciding what to wear or picking what's for dinner, might go a long way in helping them feel like themselves.

At the end of the day, the goal is to make sure they can keep living life in a way that feels like they have some control over it. With some extra support, they might be able to continue to do what they love and feel good about who they are.

Staying Strong and Balanced

You may have noticed that staying active makes a big difference for your loved one. Keeping up their strength and balance can help prevent falls, which can be a major setback. Programs that focus on building strength and teaching fall safety might be helpful. And if walking is tough, tools like walkers or adding railings around the house might help give them the support they need.

Finding Purpose

I think that independence isn't just about what they do but also about *why* they do it. When seniors feel needed or have goals to work toward, it might give them a reason to get up in the morning. Even small things, like cooking or organizing a drawer, might bring a sense of purpose for them. Volunteering for positive purposes might also be a nice way to stay active and feel useful if they're able to.

Keeping Their Memory Sharp

You might have seen how staying active, both physically and mentally, might help them stay sharp. Simple routines and little challenges, like puzzles or learning something new, might make a difference to their memory.

Nurturing Bonds

To build a good relationship with your elderly loved one, it might be important to help them stay independent. You might have already set up their/your home to make it safer, like adding railings or clearing trip hazards. Another way to help might be to introduce them to digital tools, like video calls, to stay connected with family.

Safety and Independence

Falls can be life-changing, and the stats tell that they're a major cause of injuries for seniors. You might have noticed your loved one brushing off concerns about their balance or physical changes, which might make these conversations tricky. The good news is that there can be some ways to help reduce risks without taking away their independence.

You can try to make small changes first. For example, adding a white stripe to the edge of stairs can make them easier to see, especially if your elderly loved one's vision isn't as sharp as it used to be. If your home has thick, plush carpets, you might want to consider swapping them for lower-pile options, which might help reduce tripping hazards, especially if your loved one shuffles a bit when walking.

Also, you can try to encourage your elderly loved one to

use a cane or walker. I know some seniors hesitate because they don't want to feel 'old' or stand out, but these aids can help to *protect* their independence by avoiding falls. Sometimes, it takes seeing the impact of a fall to understand the value of these tools, but it's worth encouraging them gently before it gets to that point.

Even one day spent mostly in bed can lead to some muscle loss, so staying active is important. Senior centers usually have balance and fitness classes, which can be a fun way to build strength and confidence while socializing. If they're hesitant, you might frame it as a way to stay independent longer instead of focusing on fall prevention.

You might have heard your elderly loved one say safety devices like alarms or fall detectors are unnecessary or 'for old people.' But I think these tools might give them the freedom to move around their home with a little more confidence. Remind them it's not about limiting their independence but trying to make sure they can keep doing the things they love.

You may have also already noticed your loved one saying things like, "I haven't fallen - yet." In my opinion, that little word "yet" carries so much weight. It's important to acknowledge their efforts to stay safe while gently pointing out that taking precautions *before* something happens might be the best way to stay independent.

Upholding Their Independence

Starting in-home care can feel like a big change, and you can consider it natural for your parent or elderly loved one to resist needing help. They might have spent so much of their lives managing things on their own that adjusting to having assistance might be tough. But I think that through some ways, you might be able to help them keep as much independence as possible while still getting the support they need.

Keeping Active

You may have noticed how staying active helps with strength and balance. Even gentle exercises, like walking or stretching, might make a difference. If they're up for it, resistance exercises might help rebuild and maintain muscle, which is especially important as we age. Aerobic activities, like swimming, can also boost their endurance, which might help make everyday tasks easier.

Regular movement can also do a lot, such as:

- It might help to lower the risk of heart disease, diabetes, and even some cancers.

- It might help strengthen bones to prevent fractures, especially in women after menopause.

- It might help improve mental health by reducing stress and improving confidence.

- Also, it might reduce the chances of falls, which might lead to long recoveries.

I would say that it might be never too late to get started, and the benefits might show up quickly. Even small efforts can improve their balance, coordination, and ability to handle daily routines.

You might want to start with simple steps. Encourage them to stretch in the morning, take short walks, or join a light fitness class at a senior center. If they're not willing much, remind them that these activities might help them stay strong and independent.

I think your role might be important here. You can gently

motivate them by focusing on how these activities can help them keep doing what they enjoy, like gardening, visiting friends, or even just moving around the house more easily.

Which Exercises Work Best?

The right exercises might make a difference in your elderly loved one's health, mobility, and overall independence. I think there's something for almost everyone, no matter their ability level.

The type of exercise might depend on their individual abilities, but here are some options to consider:

- Walking or hiking can be a great way for your loved one to stay active while enjoying some fresh air and sunshine.

- Swimming or water aerobics is also considered to be gentle on the joints and might work well for improving overall fitness.

- Stretching is simple but can be effective - it helps them stay flexible and eases stiffness.

- Gardening might let your elderly loved one connect with nature.

- Cycling, even at a slow pace, might help in building stamina if they're feeling up to it.

- Balance exercises can be considered important, too, especially if falls are a concern.

When you're trying to help your loved one stay active, I think it's important to keep a few things in mind. Make sure the activity matches their fitness level so it stays safe and enjoyable. And if they have medical conditions or disabilities, it's a good idea to check with their doctor before trying anything new. For those with limited mobility, gentle activities might still help - like passive exercises, where you assist with movements to keep their joints flexible, or gentle handling to keep them comfortable and encourage small movements over time.

What if Someone Has Dementia?

By now, you might have already gotten the idea that staying physically active is good, but did you know it's considered especially important for people with dementia or mild cognitive impairments?

According to a study, regular exercise over 6 to 12 months might help improve cognitive scores.[28] In my opinion, that's a big deal! And there's more – it might also be connected to how our bodies age. We talked about telomeres before, which are little "caps" at the ends of our DNA. They're like a marker for aging. Shorter telomeres are linked to diseases like dementia, cancer, and even weaker bones. Research shows that moderate aerobic exercise, like brisk walking or light cycling, for six months or more might slow down that telomere shortening.[29]

Exercise might also help the brain, too. For healthy adults, regular aerobic exercise might boost cognitive scores, which means it might help slow down cognitive decline by improving blood flow in the brain and reducing risks tied to small blood

[28] Ahlskog, J. E., Geda, Y. E., Graff-Radford, N. R., & Petersen, R. C. (2011, September). Physical exercise as a preventive or disease-modifying treatment of dementia and brain aging. In *Mayo clinic proceedings* (Vol. 86, No. 9, pp. 876-884). Elsevier.

[29] Song, S., Lee, E., & Kim, H. (2022). Does exercise affect telomere length? A systematic review and meta-analysis of randomized controlled trials. *Medicina*, 58(2), 242.

vessel issues that can lead to dementia.

Now, you might be wondering, "What about older adults who are frail or not very active right now?" A study looked at older folks who followed a simple home-based exercise routine paired with good nutrition.[30] The results were that they improved their physical abilities and even scored better on frailty measures.

And let's not forget that staying active doesn't have to mean big gym workouts. Even small, consistent movements, fit to your loved one's abilities, might make a difference. Plus, there are apps and online tools that can guide and encourage physical activity. These e-health strategies might be a good option if you're looking for easy, accessible ways to help your loved one stay active.

Independence can be considered a major part of dignity and happiness, especially for our elderly loved ones. Supporting their independence doesn't mean doing everything for them, but I think it's rather about finding ways to help them stay involved in their own care and routines. After all, a little encouragement and understanding might go a long way in helping them maintain an active life!

---

[30] Hsieh, T. J., Su, S. C., Chen, C. W., Kang, Y. W., Hu, M. H., Hsu, L. L., ... & Hsu, C. C. (2019). Individualized home-based exercise and nutrition interventions improve frailty in older adults: a randomized controlled trial. *International Journal of Behavioral Nutrition and Physical Activity*, *16*, 1-15.

Chapter 13: The Importance of Social Engagement in Later Life

How many times have you found yourself in a situation where you needed someone you could talk to — someone you could confide in or even someone whose presence would mean something, even if neither of you spoke a word? It is in the very nature of human beings to build connections, as those connections provide us with the strength to navigate through the rough waters of life. Besides, we, as human beings, are social animals who thrive on the basis of bonds and relations. Since it is innate, therefore, every individual needs to build social connections no matter what their age may be. Isolating one's self and connecting you is simply against human nature.

People in their old age are more prone to developing various ailments — both mental and physical, with depression being on top of the list. According to recent research, depression is proven to be one of the underlying causes of dementia. While depression is one of the significant mental health issues, there are several psychological issues that may result in the absence of a social connection or a bond. Individuals, regardless of their age, require building bonds as such keep them motivated to do better in their lives. Such being the case, how important do you think building a social repertoire of relations would be for the elderly? Before we establish the significance of that in the lives of senior people, it is essential to understand and grasp a fair picture of what an ordinary would be like for people of old age.

Challenges that come with a lack of Social Connection

Let's face it, they don't have much to do and life just continues to go on and on for those around them while they fade in the backdrop of life quietly day after day until they breathe their last. This might make you want to ask, isn't it what old age is all about? Of course, it is. However, fading away quietly, becoming invisible to those around them, tends to do more damage than one can imagine. Why do you think that people of a certain age are prone to diseases, the underlying cause of which is, more often than not, isolation? This is because while those around them, be it their children or any caregivers, get caught up in the seemingly impossible tangle of an impossibly busy life, these senior citizens do not have many people they can talk to.

Imagine sitting all by yourself and not having a single soul around you to talk to, or even utter a single word — and this, by the way, becomes a norm for you — your everyday life. How would you take it? It will take a toll on your mental health, don't you think? If you, being a healthy individual, tend to lose your sanity if you are made to be isolated, how do you think it is going to play out for those who are no less like children? What is, after all, old age, if not regression, in terms of your health, both mental and physiological? This is just one aspect of addressing the importance of social bonding in the lives of seniors. Social

Significance of Social Connection

Isolation can also result in premature death for the elderly while becoming the root cause of several chronic illnesses. Not only are people of a certain age group, in this case, the elderly, becoming more prone to terminal diseases, but they may also experience cardiac arrest due to a lack of social connectedness. While people of this age group develop Type-2 diabetes because of being caught up in an endless cycle of isolation, these people also become suicidal without even realizing it. Keeping yourself from interacting with people can be devastating for your mental health. Once your mental health is affected, your entire body begins to give up. That's when your body parts stop functioning to their full capacity. This happens naturally to anyone who stays out of touch with other individuals, especially in terms of communication. While individuals ranging from the age of 5 to 40 are more equipped in terms of their health to survive the aftereffects of depression, the elderly have no such benefit. Instead, they become weak. Their health deteriorates by the day. It is, therefore, quite essential for people of this age group to have a social standing, preventing them from falling into the darkest pits of isolation.

Being socially active and continuing to engage with people is one of the most important aspects of ageing rather healthily — mentally as well as physically. Now, this might make you wonder how social engagement helps age healthily. The answer is quite simple, really. When you know you are involved and valued in a gathering, it makes you want to be there. You not only make plans, but you act on them. This itself ensures that you do not stay confined to the walls of your living space and instead, make efforts to leave that confinement and be physically present where you are required to be.

Stepping out of your comfort zone will, in turn, allow you to leave behind your reservations and mingle with people. One thing that becomes a constant when you reach your old age is isolation, which leads you to overanalyze your surroundings. Before you know it, you find yourself tangled in the deep web of depression. Besides, it is a well-established fact that social interactions, building bonds, and social connectedness not only influence your overall living experience but also enable you to do better every day.

Turning old means dealing with a long list of challenges that may seem a far-off dream when you are still young but that far-off dream becomes an everyday reality for you once you are old. This list of challenges includes retirement, a life without those you loved because of their demise, and not being able to move physically as freely as you could back in the day. Now, with these many challenges, something easily creeps up into your life. You lose touch with almost everyone. It is not something you do to yourself voluntarily; it just naturally happens.

When a lack of interaction creeps into your life, you are ultimately left to face many mental health challenges. This is why, though it cannot be emphasized enough, establishing connections and ensuring they continue to exist is highly essential for people of all ages— but most importantly, the elderly. Being socially involved gives senior people a sense of belonging and purpose, which adds to the significance of social connectedness in the lives of people of old age.

Impact of Social Connection on Mental Health

While the positive impact social connectedness has on the elderly is seen and observed, it has also been proven by research that engaging socially helps slow down the process of cognitive decline due to old age. As a result, the chances of developing depression and anxiety are reduced to a significant extent, enhancing an individual's overall mental health, especially in old age. Apart from that, social connection impacts positively on mental health in several ways, some of which are addressed below.

Alleviating the Root Cause of Dementia

In order to minimize loneliness, which can be particularly common in older persons, social ties play an essential role in preserving emotional health. This helps reduce the chances of senior individuals developing depression, which has been proven by research to be one of the factors that could lead to dementia. Participating in community events and interacting with loved ones provide priceless companionship and emotional support, providing a sense of belonging. Through these exchanges, people can exchange ideas, sentiments, and experiences, strengthening bonds and a sense of belonging. In addition to improving mood, positive social interaction also helps people feel more a part of the world and have a higher sense of purpose.

People are more likely to feel happy, fulfilled, and stable when they feel connected to others—all of which are critical for mental health. Also, maintaining these social connections can significantly lower the risk of feeling depressed and anxious, acting as an umbrella against the emotional challenges that often accompany aging. By cultivating these relationships and taking part in social activities, the elderly can improve their overall health and quality of life.

Enhanced Cognitive Functions

People in their old age have to face challenges when it comes to their memory retention and cognitive function. However, their cognitive abilities significantly improve when they develop and maintain strong social bonds. Social interaction improves general mental health by stimulating several brain functions in addition to offering friendship. Regular social engagement has been shown to increase brain activity and either postpone or lower the risk of dementia and

Alzheimer's disease. These encounters, whether through meaningful talks, group activities, or community events, stimulate the brain and promote mental acuity. Seniors can actively strive toward preserving their cognitive health and leading more satisfying lives by placing a higher priority on social interaction.

Building social contacts provides seniors with a channel to let their inner thoughts flow and be able to express their emotions, worries, and frustrations in a more nurturing atmosphere. They are able to talk about difficulties they confront and share personal experiences when they have meaningful conversations with others, whether those people be friends, family, or classmates. More so, to relieve their emotional weight, this interaction garners a feeling of community and belonging.

Stabilized Regulation of Emotions

Social interactions provide senior individuals with a chance to think about their feelings, which is important for processing emotions. They can feel validated in their experiences by talking about their concerns or frustrations with someone who understands and listens. This sympathetic relationship can greatly lessen the sense of loneliness that is frequently experienced by seniors.

When you start sharing your thoughts with people around you, you, as a senior individual, will be surprised to see how it can lead to remarkable results, such as providing you with insightful counsel or alternative viewpoints. This enables you, as well as those around you, to handle the circumstances more skillfully. Besides, when there is a decrease in levels of stress, emotional burdens are effortlessly lifted. This promotes mental clarity and establishes mental stability. Ultimately, building resilience and advancing general emotional well-being depends on having a support system where people feel heard and valued.

Help in Preventing a Sense of Stagnancy

It can, most of the time, get exasperating to be in the same routine, especially if it becomes a norm — something that you do every day as if it is a part of a constant running loop. You are naturally inclined to feel a sense of stagnancy which may make you feel irritated, leading you to develop a need for breaking this cycle. Now, this is something that can happen to people of all ages. However, it is much more challenging for people of old age, given that they do not have much on their hands to cater to. Their routine simply revolves around waking up, watching the day unfold, going back to sleep, and repeating it all over again for the days that are to follow. As a result of this, senior citizens become prone to depression, which can get worse by reaching a stage where isolation becomes their comfort zone. This is extremely unhealthy for older people.

Social connectedness helps them break this cycle by providing them with something new every day. Once senior people find themselves becoming an integral part of society, they break free of the stagnancy that they may not initially be able to identify. Since social interactions require you to jog your brain in order to produce more ideas and exchange those ideas with others, you naturally come out of the state of being stagnant. Besides, building social bonds is not limited to enhancing one's mental health. What you need to understand here is that while engaging with those around you helps you become a better version of yourself, especially in old age, it is also, at the same time, building a more substantial, much more diversified community where ideas stemming from distinct minds are shared.

How Involvement in Community Helps

The elderly can feel like important and contributing members of society by continuing to be involved in the community. There is a long list of things the elderly can resort to in order to keep themselves occupied within the community. This includes volunteering, joining clubs, and attending neighborhood activities. When old age individuals find themselves involved, Seniors who participate in the community have the chance to learn new skills, take up hobbies, or rekindle interests that they may have put aside during their working years. This will help them build a routine for themselves, allowing them to avoid isolating themselves altogether.

Why Social Connectedness Becomes Essential in Old Age

As we grow and transition into our older years, the importance of connections becomes even more essential than it ever can be. During this phase of life, friendships and peer interactions become an integral part of emotional well-being, even if family ties usually remain strong. These connections go much beyond simple friendship; even when we face the difficulties of age, they provide priceless emotional support, create a deep sense of belonging, and generate exciting chances for personal development.

The elderly, more often than not, experience a decrease in social interactions as they get older and retire. Daily routines that were discussed above, mainly working, raising kids, or pursuing a career, often disappear, creating a gap in social interaction chances. Feelings of loneliness may result from this change, and it seems sense that loneliness could become a serious issue at this time. But it is of grave importance to keep in mind that making and maintaining friendships can be quite advantageous. These relationships can bridge the gap by offering the emotional support and sense of purpose that are so essential for our well-being as we age.

Having friends later in life helps provide a special kind of emotional support. Bonds weaved out of friendships are characteristically more deep-rooted than interactions with family members, which may come with duties or expectations. Friends provide empathy, support, and frequently a feeling of commonality. Seniors may feel more at ease sharing personal details with those people who are experiencing comparable life transitions, such as retirement, health issues, or the death of a spouse. This mutual comprehension creates strong emotional bonds that are good for mental wellness.

Closing Thoughts

Building and nurturing social connections in later life can significantly affect the emotional health of those who reach their old age. Acknowledging the value of peer connections allows us to see how they offer essential companionship, support, and chances for personal development.

Group activities and senior centers can be friendly places for seniors to make new friends, take part in meaningful activities, and form enduring relationships. Seniors who engage in these social activities not only fight loneliness but also maintain mental and physical activity, which gives them a sense of fulfillment and purpose in their later years. It's encouraging to know that making new friends is never impossible and that their emotional depth can genuinely improve one's quality of life.

Part V:
Supporting the Supporters

Chapter 14: Before You Can Give, Take Care

Being a caregiver puts a lot of responsibilities on your shoulders, not to mention that it is no easy feat because of the challenges that come with it. While it may be one of the most beautiful feelings in the world to take care of those who, in worse worst-case scenario, forget their names, it is undeniably a task only a man of strong character and wit can handle. It is a responsibility that puts you to the test and trial, not just physically but emotionally and mentally as well.

Are you, as a caregiver, ready to take up the difficulties that come with it? While it may seem to be an act of kindness and your contribution to society, are you strong enough to let your patience be put to the test? That's food for thought for the readers, the answer to which you will be better able to provide once you understand what it feels like to be a caregiver.

This chapter will not only highlight the role of a caregiver, sketching a complete picture of their life and what a typical day in their life looks like, but will also provide the readers with an insight as to who qualifies as a caregiver and what it takes to be one. In this chapter, while you navigate through the ins and outs of a dementia patient's caregiver, you will also be introduced to ways in which caregivers can ensure their well-being, both mentally and physically, as they provide their nurturing to those who unknowingly suffer from the aftermath of dementia and other illnesses that fall under its canopy.

Before we delve deeper into further details pertaining to the life of a caregiver, it is essential for the readers to understand what it means to be a caregiver and how an individual qualifies to be one.

What Does It Mean by a Caregiver?

A caregiver is someone who takes care of you — you could be anyone who needs nurturing and someone to be around you almost all the time so that you don't end up hurting yourself in any way. In the context of dementia, individuals who suffer significant memory loss cannot be left alone on their own because they are constantly at risk of coming in harm's way. Now, a caregiver can be anyone; it can be a professional, a family member, a distant relative, or even an individual who chooses to volunteer for a task as significant as taking care of those who are in dire need of your assistance 24/7.

What one must understand here is that such a task is not limited to watching over someone. It is an act that requires you to adjust your life according to those who are under their care. So, I ask you again, do you think of yourself as someone capable enough to not only allow your patience to be put to the test but also mold your schedule in accordance with an individual who may not have any clue about their lives whatsoever? It requires skill, but more than that, it requires you to be steadfast even when the situation tends to get challenging, potentially taking a toll on you emotionally. Understand that caregivers can be one of the following:

From Flesh and Blood to Caregivers

Your flesh and blood, your family members, are those people who know you better than anyone else, even if, with time, you have become distant. Family members, including your spouse, children, grandchildren, siblings, parents, and grandparents, can be amongst the best caregivers one can ever ask for. They not only know when you need what, but they also understand your needs even without you saying a word about them.

Understand here that dementia and chronic diseases that fall under the umbrella of dementia make it quite challenging for an individual to take care of themselves on their own. Under such circumstances, a member of the family, your very own kith and kin can evidently be the most favorable option to be chosen as a caregiver. While people may have or have not such an option due to various reasons, the role of taking care of someone who's grown too old to look after themselves, often naturally falls on a loved one. This is primarily because you grow in their presence, and even if there is no word uttered, being a part of the same blood makes you understand a lot about one another naturally. It is more like an innate radar that instinctively picks on anything that is different than usual, something that does not align with the *normal* dynamics of anyone among the kin.

Of course, there are professional caregivers who can be hired for such a demanding job. They would undoubtedly do a remarkable job at that because they would be paid for it, and it's their job. So sure, they would be a great option. However, what your loved ones do for you is entirely out of love and the responsibility they hold towards you. It may not even be their responsibility, but they do it out of commitment and even necessity sometimes.

How a member of the family sees it as a responsibility is in accordance with the reciprocal of the care. When a child is born, it is under the constant care of the parents until the child turns of a certain age. When a parent encounters a chronic disease as critical as dementia, looking after them with a sense of reciprocating the same love and care does good not only to the one who's been taking care of them but also to the one looking after them. It is a bond weaved out of love and affection for one another, and in the midst of this exchange, the patient gets the best treatment and care one can get.

Nonetheless, there are times when the blood relations cannot do the needful and there comes the option of a professional caregiver. There are various reasons why your own blood and flesh may not be able to be there for you in times as difficult as suffering from a chronic disease. One of these reasons may include not having enough time because of the hustle-bustle of life.

It is a known fact — a new normal for people to start their day already rushing through their daily tasks, struggling to get things done within the span of a day to not let it add to the pile of pending work. Earning money requires people to show up at work, or even if you are working remotely, you still need to be actively working as some tasks require your 100% participation. While you find yourself juggling one task and another, it becomes nearly impossible for you to be there for loved ones, especially when they cannot look after themselves.

When you cannot do it on your own, there is no shame in getting someone hired to take care of elderly people suffering from dementia or Alzheimer's disease. There are several benefits of hiring professionals to be by the patient's side 24/7 without having to risk anything since their job is to be present with the patient. Before we address what, the potential benefits are of hiring a professional caregiver, let's first understand the ins and outs of a professional caregiver.

Who Qualifies as a Professional Caregiver?

While it may seem a one-person job, it has been observed that taking care of a patient with Alzheimer's disease or dementia requires a team of people and may not be the job of a single soul. This is because of various reasons. At times, it becomes difficult to handle the patient single-handedly. One can keep an eye on the patient while the other prepares the meal or preps the dose of medication. In this collaborative setting, the chances of making an error, which may result in fatality, are reduced significantly. Professionally, every person has a distinctive job when it comes to providing care.

Understand that every individual professionally responsible for taking care of people suffering from dementia has to play a distinct role. Providing thorough care for someone who not only keeps forgetting essential details pertaining to their lives but also fails to explain their basic needs and feelings requires not one but multiple minds. It is not to be taken as a job for one man. Also, in a more professional setting, the need for a team of caregivers roots from each person having specialized skills. One may be exceptionally good at reinforcing memories for a patient with dementia but may not be as good in helping them perform their day-to-day task.

When it comes to professional caregivers, the people involved are mainly the nurses, in-home care providers, palliative or hospice caregivers and doctors as well.

In-home Caregivers: these are the professionals who are hired to help people with dementia perform their basic functions like eating, bathing, taking medicines, and reminding patients of their names, relations, and faces. These home aides usually visit houses, providing basic care, attending to the patient's basic necessities, keeping them occupied with small chores while staying with the patient all the time. These professionals may work for half a day or a full day, depending on their shift hours. While they may relieve you of the worry of providing constant attention for your loved ones who suffer from dementia, they may not be equipped to provide advanced medical assistance. That's where the option of nurses lies.

Nurses: there are individuals who attain certification in nursing and provide services that require a much-advanced form of caregiving. These nurses could be at home or could perform their duties within the walls of a nursing home, ensuring the well-being of patients suffering from Alzheimer's disease or other underlying causes of dementia. These individuals require certification in this field that ensures that they are qualified enough to attend to duties such as administrating medications, tending to the wounds that patients acquire quite regularly due to decline in their cognitive abilities and monitoring symptoms and acting accordingly. In a situation where the circumstances reach a point where there's nothing much that could be done to save the patient, then such circumstances demand someone who can ensure making patients comfortable as they near the end of their time. When the hour arrives when there's nothing a nurse can do to alleviate the symptoms, hospice or palliative care providers come into play.

Resting Home or Palliative Care Providers: there are times when the patients reach a point where there is nothing that can be done to save them. They reach the final stage of their illness, where the only thing that can be done is to make them feel comfortable as they drift gradually to the realm of death, leaving behind the land of the living.

When such times arrive, the best care these patients can get is companionship, someone who can make them understand that they are not alone and help them provide as much comfort as lies in their power. While palliative caregivers could be limited for those who are on the verge of death, there are volunteers who work not only as palliative workers but are also happy to do every job that falls under their scope of skills when it comes to providing thorough care for patients with dementia.

Volunteers: these people work out of the goodness of their hearts in the name of social work, with a mindset of contributing to the well-being of society as a whole. There are organizations and social groups who strive to make the world a better place and, in their endeavor, to do so, they send their people to places where help is required. Now, help can come in several forms, and providing care for those who have forgotten their identity, their loved ones, and the life they had is one of those forms of help.

Volunteers provide their assistance by offering transport for these people taking care of the patients part-time or full-time as per their availability. In best-case scenarios, these volunteers offer to spend their time with those elderly who fall behind in life due to a decline in their cognitive functions. The most important thing that the elderly need in their life is someone they can spend their time with, alleviating their ever-increasing loneliness.

While volunteers, as a contribution to society, offer their time to anyone who tends to feel left behind, they are exceptionally good at taking care of people with dementia. In their eyes, it's a contribution to society. Now that we know who qualifies as a caregiver, it is essential to understand what responsibilities lie on the shoulders of a care provider, whether the individual is a professional or a loved one.

The Role of a Caregiver

Do you think taking care of the individuals with dementia is an easy feat? To understand the role and responsibility of a caregiver, it is essential to remember the difference between dementia and Alzheimer's disease. While dementia serves as an umbrella term for those diseases that affect a person's memory and cognitive ability, Alzheimer's disease serves as one of the many causes of dementia and a major one at that.

Once you know the difference, it becomes easy for you to sketch a picture of the responsibilities that come with providing care for patients who suffer memory loss in general, while other symptoms may vary depending on the type or cause of dementia. A caregiver is responsible for keeping an eye on the patient whose cognitive abilities are impaired with time due to underlying causes. It is to be understood that the role of a caregiver goes above and beyond mere assistance in daily tasks. It requires a lot more than just providing help with day-to-day activities. The list goes as follows:

Constant Reminders

It is one of the major responsibilities of a caregiver to provide constant reminders to those who suffer from diseases that fall under the canopy of dementia, Alzheimer's being one of them. When a person encounters such a condition, it does not show overnight but develops with time. People with dementia, primarily Alzheimer's disease, experience cognitive decline leading to memory loss. Due to this, the patient tends to forget names, faces, relations, and events that a person with no such disease or condition may never forget.

It is one of the key roles of a caregiver to repeatedly remind the patient of the names, faces, relations, and events that hold special importance in the patient's life. While reminding someone of something that they keep forgetting over and over again may be emotionally exhausting for the caregiver, a caregiver is essentially responsible for reinforcing memories that keep leaving the patient's mind.

Helping Navigate Communication

Dementia causes a decline in one's cognitive ability. When such is the case, it is only natural for the patient to experience disorientation because of which communication becomes difficult. Since the patient's memory tends to take a hit due to such chronic diseases that fall under dementia, this is suggestive of the idea — and has also been observed — that a patient starts to forget words and form sentences.

This makes it difficult for the patient to relay a message as simple as feeling thirsty. This is because when there is a decline in their memory, the patients are unable to give names to their condition and feelings. It falls on the shoulders of a caregiver to come up with ways to promote communication.

While reinforcing information is essential, methods used to reinforce information are more significant, requiring them to be effective, regardless of how simple or complex the methods are. In order to help patients with Alzheimer's disease and others that cause dementia, reinforce the use of visual aids, non-verbal cues and instill the use of language that is simple, easier to understand, and remember using words that are not complex and are rather straightforward.

Managing Behaviors:

People suffering from dementia are more likely to experience changes in their moods and behavior. This change occurs quite repeatedly, as a result of which the patient becomes weary of their own tempers. In situations where this tends to escalate, it is the job of a caregiver to ensure that the patient's mood is regulated in accordance with the need of the hour. When the patient experiences irritability and becomes aggressive which is quite possible in cases of dementia, a caregiver is responsible for making the patient navigate through such moods and temperaments.

More so, it is observed quite commonly that patients who suffer from dementia are more prone to anxiety than any other individual who does not display symptoms of any sort of mental illness, let alone Alzheimer's disease. It is seen that these patients can experience heightened levels of anxiety, which may occur in the form of extreme fear or relentlessness. Another sign that a patient with dementia displays of anxiety could be irritability.

Patients with dementia often show signs of paranoia, and keeping them calm and relaxed is not something anyone can pull. It requires a lot of patience and strong-headedness to keep the patients' anxiety from not only elevating but also transitioning into a panic attack. Caregivers, with their love, patience, and resilience, can ensure that when patients feel elevated levels of anxiety, they have in front of their eyes a face that provides a sense of familiarity, making their job all the more challenging.

The Challenges that come with Caregiving

What happens when the tables are turned, and the caregiver ends up needing the care? Do you think providing care and looking after someone who keeps forgetting everything and has to be reminded of basics is something anyone can do? The job of a caregiver, whether the caregiver is a professional or a loved one, requires a lot of patience. There are times when the provider ends up needing to be at the receiving end. This is because there are several challenges that come their way while fulfilling their duties. Here's a list of challenges that a caregiver is likely to encounter.

Physical Strain and Exhaustion

Caring for someone can be challenging in so many ways, physical strain being one of them. It requires you, as a caregiver, to follow the patients wherever they go in order to ensure their safety. There are times when patients with dementia may need physical assistance, like helping them get up from their bed, take a walk, sit in a wheelchair, etc. There are times when patients with dementia are required to perform physical exercise, like taking a stroll or doing simple chores to keep the body moving.

These are the tasks that people with dementia cannot be left to do on their own. When a caregiver attends to their patients, it is only natural for them to feel exhausted and physically strained. More so, there are chances that lifting and moving the patients from one to another may cause muscle sprain. In the worst-case scenario, physical exhaustion may lead to long-term medical issues.

Emotional Toll

At some point, the responsibilities that come with taking care of a patient with dementia tend to have an emotional toll on you. Patients with Alzheimer's disease or any other form of dementia are not in their normal state of mind. Their minds are not functioning like generally their minds would. There is a significant decline in their cognitive functions leading them to do things that may not only be detrimental to them but may push the caregivers to a point of exasperation.

No matter how patient and resilient you are when your patience is put to the test constantly, you are likely to snap, and such a response is only natural. Nonetheless, the caregiver may find themselves losing their calm by the day till the point where they begin to believe they don't have it in them anymore. This may result in a caregiver developing mental issues like depression.

Time Management

Being a caregiver requires you to sacrifice a massive chunk of your time, leaving you with little to no time for yourself. Whether you are a professional, a loved one, or even a volunteer, you will find yourself in a time rush, with you have not enough time on your hands to cater to your personal life. Your social life may also suffer greatly because your hours are spent taking care of someone who is suffering from dementia. How can you be able to do something else when more than half of your day is spent taking care of someone else? This may make you, as a caregiver, feel like you do not have a life of your own. While it may make you feel better for helping someone who cannot look after themselves without you, not having to do something that adds value to yourself personally tends to make you feel unfulfilled.

Lack of Skillset

No matter how much you love them, you DO NOT possess the answer to every question there is in the book. Understand that not everybody can do everything, and when it comes to taking care of those who cannot even perform basic functions. Patients with dementia fail to perform activities such as leaving the bed and remembering to come back or voicing out their feelings, pain, and emotions. This makes it difficult for the caregiver, if the caregiver is not a professional, to understand what can be done to help the patient.

Financial Issues

Taking care of patients who suffer from chronic conditions such as dementia requires you to pay a huge sum of money. You are not only paying the bills of the hospital and medications, but you are also paying for a lot of things that people with dementia may need constantly. Looking after someone with declining mental and physical health is financially challenging. You may not be able to afford proper care for the patient as you may have already spent a massive amount of money already. This can leave you in debt, and you may not be able to send the patient to a nursing home — a private one — since they charge you huge sums of money.

Looking after patients with dementia challenges you in almost every aspect of your life. Your physical health tends to take a toll. You get exhausted not just physically but mentally as well. You may experience difficulty navigating through financial crises. You will end up feeling an exasperating sense of unfulfillment. All this can be dealt with if you, as a caregiver, allow yourself to be taken care of.

When a Caregiver Needs Care

There are times when tables can turn, and a caregiver may end up needing care, which, by the way, is not only natural but also essential. There are several options available for you to find help when you are in dire need of it. What you need to understand here is that life is not easy for anyone and you are not the only one needing help. This is not to make you feel bad about needing some extra hand to help you through your journey as a caregiver but to tell you that it is okay to ask for help when you need it. There is no shame in asking for support when things start to get out of your hands. Here is what you can do:

1. Expect what's real. Do not allow yourself to fall prey to unrealistic expectations that since you are a caregiver so, you magically know everything. You don't. There will be challenges and it is only wise to expect them and not ignore their existence. You need to be mindful of the fact that you are not someone know-it-all, so there will be things you won't be able to do. That's completely okay. Be kind to yourself when you find yourself not doing something in its perfect form.

2. Ask for help. It cannot be emphasized enough that you will only get help when you ask for it. No one is capable of reading your mind. While you may be dying inside and, your face may deceive others into thinking that you are absolutely fine. Let people know you need them. Do not be embarrassed to ask people when you need their help.

3. Sure, you earn a sufficient amount of money, but there is no need to go bankrupt when you know you will not be able to take care of a patient with dementia in the long run. The best way to deal with financial constraints is to opt for organizations that provide assistance for free. Using government-run facilities also serves as a good option when your financial limitations keep you from taking care of your loved ones.

4. Take a break because you need it! You do not have to take long hours of break to break free from the exhaustive cycle of providing thorough care. Taking small breaks will help you from reaching a point of exhaustion where you cannot function at all.

5. Use self-help books. They are your friend. Reading and educating yourself on this matter will help you

understand more, allowing you as ease of navigation through the challenges of providing care for patients with dementia.

6. Set boundaries not just for others but for yourself as well. Set realistic targets and stick to them. Make it a boundary for yourself to not overdo something that may drain you entirely.

Bottomline

While caregivers may be the ones responsible for looking after patients suffering from dementia, it is the responsibility of society as a whole to take care of those who nurture such patients. This is essential for their well-being because if they are not taken care of well, in turn attending to patients with dementia, then there is a likelihood of them falling prey to mental illnesses.

Chapter 15: United in Caring

You do not have to do this alone. One person may be handling it well, but it is never a one-person job. You can have a team of caregivers. It is a generalized idea that when it comes to taking care of someone suffering from a chronic disease such as dementia, there is one person in the family who shoulders the burden of taking care of the sick. It does not have to be that way. It is not a rule or a law that only one person has to bear the responsibility of looking after a patient with dementia. A team of two or more people can do a remarkable job when it comes to looking after a sick person, especially if they are facing challenges pertaining to their cognitive abilities. While the idea may seem absurd and alienating, it is not, and in fact, it serves better than one soul handling it all on their own.

Collaborative Caregiving: Understanding Teamwork

Understanding what collective caregiving is essential before we explore other areas under collective caregiving or teamwork in caregiving. It is often observed that when an individual falls sick in which that individual suffers a drastic decline in their cognitive abilities, family members step in to look after that individual. Now, it is natural to assume that given the fast-paced life, we have these days, the member of the family who has time on their hands step up and take responsibility. While this may be the case with most families, there are times when other family members do not shy away from playing a part in a task as challenging and as significant as taking care of the elderly who are unable to lead a normal life due to dementia.

While it has been discussed before in the previous chapters, it is essential for the readers to remember what dementia is because knowing the issue to its deepest core is the only way to resolve it. It is only fair to keep an emphasis on the difference between dementia and other chronic diseases that affect an individual's cognitive abilities such as reasoning, retaining information, making perceptions, evaluating a situation, etc. primarily where memory is affected, the individual is said to have an ailment that falls under the canopy of dementia. Dementia is an umbrella term — a set of symptoms where there is a significant decline in one's ability to retain information and act in accordance with that information. While dementia is a set of these symptoms, Alzheimer's disease is one of the many causes of dementia. This allows the reader to have a sound understanding of what the root cause is, enabling them to do a better, more profound job when it comes to looking after individuals who suffer from these fateful symptoms. One thing that is common in all types of dementia is deteriorating memory.

Now that we have established what the main illness is, it becomes easier here to develop a sense of understanding about collective caregiving and how it can be woven to make the living experience better for the patients who suffer memory loss, are unable to perform the day-to-day task on their own and navigate through the exasperating pathways of isolation and a sense of being lost.

What is Collective/Collaborative Caregiving?

Collective or collaborative caregiving refers to two or more people teaming up to make themselves available to attend to the needs of a patient who suffers from a chronic condition. In this case, that chronic condition is Alzheimer's disease and symptoms that point towards the onset of dementia. To understand collaborative caregiving and the purpose of this teamwork, it is essential to acknowledge the fact that people suffering from chronic diseases that affect their memory require well-rounded attention to be taken care of every hour of the day. This is because their cognitive ability experiences a drastic decline, making it nearly impossible for such patients to perform even the most trivial tasks one can think of.

Collaborative or collective caregiving is a method of providing comprehensive care to patients who show signs of dementia. Here, multiple individuals team up in order to ensure that not only does the patient receive thorough care and attention around the clock but also feels whole emotionally. In patients with dementia, it is quite commonly observed that their mental health tends to take a toll. They may not be able to remember names, faces, and relations and lose track of time, but the realization that they cannot remember something tends to make them feel agitated. This can lead to several mental health challenges, including anxiety, depression, and, in some cases, paranoia. When a patient suffering from dementia has a team of caregivers and not just one person looking after them, it becomes a smoother process for the patient as well as the caregiver to make life a better, much more bearable experience for the patient and those around them.

Apart from the patient's point of view, it is highly essential for us to understand why collaborative care helps not just the patient but the caregiver as well.

Helping the Helper

Understand that taking care of someone whose reasoning, the ability to retain information and act rationally is impaired is no easy job and can more often than not affect the health of

216

those who volunteer to take care of such people. While it may initially just wear the caregiver down, such a job is undeniably exhausting mentally, too. It is, therefore, quite essential for those individuals who sign up for such a task to have someone by their side so that this entire process does not become overwhelming. Collaborative caregiving can help not just the patients but also the ones in charge of looking after those patients.

What makes living a difficult experience for those suffering from dementia is the nature of this condition. Since such a condition progresses with time, the simple, day-to-day tasks become impossible for patients to perform on their own. These tasks may include eating, taking medicines timely, bathing, and getting dressed. While an individual can and does help a patient with dementia with all such activities, a collaborative initiative ensures that these activities are well-administered and the risk of failing to meet the requirements of a caregiver is reduced. Besides, these responsibilities become manageable.

Since dementia is a condition that progresses with time, the patient becomes more and more dependent on the caregiver, leaving little to no room for the caregiver to have a moment to breathe, making this whole job a tiresome process. Having multiple people team up to help a patient with dementia with everyday activities such as eating, bathing, exercising, taking medications, and all other basic functions can make it easier for both the patient as well the one providing care. The dependency may continue to grow with time, but having multiple people looking after you can help make things easier, reducing the risk of getting both parties involved from getting affected negatively. Collaborative caregiving helps regulate responsibilities by dividing them among the group of people who sign up for such a hectic and demanding job.

Needs of a Patient with Dementia

Caregiving, whether provided by a single individual or a team of multiple individuals, can be challenging in ways unimaginable due to the needs of those who develop conditions such as Alzheimer's. It is, therefore, quite essential for us to understand what are the actual, practical needs of those suffering from dementia. The first thing that experiences a hit when a person begins to develop dementia or the disease starts to show its onset is a decline in memory.

Losing one's memory and having difficulty not only recalling something from the past but also retaining information is a key element of dementia and other diseases that fall under dementia. As the condition advances, the patient finds it difficult and sometimes even impossible to remember anything. Initially, it is just small, insignificant things that the patient forgets. This may include not being able to remember why they entered a room where they kept their things like glasses, keys, or medicines. As the disease advances, the patients tend to experience severe brain fog, not being able to remember people's names as well as their own. When the situation gets worse, the patient completely forgets about themselves as well as their close ones. That's where a caregiver can come forward to help the patient with remembering things that the patient keeps forgetting. This is one of the issues that patients with dementia experience.

One of the major issues that patients with dementia experience other than memory loss is difficulty in communicating their needs. While this may be rooted in their inability to retain information and difficulty in remembering what they already know, they sometimes cannot put their finger on the underlying issue. As a result, the patient tends to lose their calm and may end up creating a fuss about it. This is where regulation of their mood becomes a problem, which again is something the caregiver is expected to help the patient navigate through. Finding it almost impossible to express what they are feeling can make the patients suffering from dementia lose their calm. This is one of the underlying causes of such patients experiencing mental health issues, such as anxiety, depression, and feelings of isolation. The job of a caregiver here is to ensure the patient is able to find the right words to express what's bothering the patient.

Helping patients with dementia learn to communicate again is just like teaching a baby to speak, with a few exceptions. While a child's mind develops with time as the child continues to learn more, the mind of a patient with dementia tends to deteriorate with time until there is no more room left for deterioration, and the inevitable is left where the only thing that can be done for the patient is to make them feel as much comfortable as possible till the time, they breathe their last — hence, the inevitable.

One of the most common observations in patients with dementia includes their rapidly changing moods. Regulation of mood in patients suffering from dementia is a task not for someone who lacks patience. It requires you to be patient enough to a point where the patient's aggression, confusion, frustration, and constantly changing moods do not get to you. Do you think you, as a caregiver, have it in you to deal with someone unwearyingly who feels one thing and another the very next moment? Think again!

It all roots from a decline in the patient's cognitive functions. Imagine you can't seem to remember your name. The person standing next to you is someone who claims to know you, but you can't recall seeing them before. There is something you feel physically, but you are unaware of ways to voice it out. There is something going on in your head, but you do not know what that is. You just know that something is happening, but you can't put your finger on it. How would you feel about all those things that are aforementioned? It is only natural for anyone to feel like they are losing their mind if they find themselves in a similar situation. When this happens, you are most likely to feel several emotions building up within you, making it all the more exasperating for you — making you feel like you are in a place of oblivion where nothing makes sense. Here's when a caregiver can provide assistance, making it possible for the patient to feel not only safe but also give the patient a sense of belonging. Such a task may be performed by one individual, but this should not be a burden for a single soul to shoulder.

Apart from constantly changing moods and a state of confusion, patients suffering from dementia can encounter difficulty catering to basic activities that do not require much hard work or knowledge. These activities have been mentioned over and over again in the text, and rightfully so. Imagine being a grown-up but not knowing how to eat something. During the onset of dementia, one of the most common symptoms is forgetting the basic knowledge that becomes a part of nature as you grow up. For example, eating food when you feel hungry.

Dementia prevents you from being able to consume food or even reach out for water when your throat runs dry. In fact, when this happens, patients with dementia tend to find themselves in a state of confusion because they can neither explain nor even understand what they are feeling, nor do they know what they are supposed to do when they feel a certain way. While eating is one of these basic activities that patients who suffer from dementia experience difficulty carrying out, bathing and getting dressed becomes just another impossible task on their list, leading them further into the darkness of the unknown. Since such patients cannot rely on themselves for ingestion, it is only natural to expect nothing from these individuals when it comes to administrating their medicines. That's where those who volunteer to look after such individuals can come forward and provide their assistance. However, this should not be the responsibility of just one individual.

Your role as a caregiver is to ensure that patients with dementia have constant assistance when they need it. Nut that assistance is not limited to just physical activity. Those who take up this noble task are also expected to provide emotional support to patients with dementia.

Advantages of Collaborative Caregiving

There are many advantages to collaborative caregiving, especially when it comes to caring for persons who have dementia. Family members, friends, and professionals can share the duties and emotional strain of providing care thanks to this team-based approach.

More Support, Less Burden

When two or more people team up to provide care and assistance for those suffering from dementia, the burden is not left for one person to shoulder. It is essential for you to understand that providing care for patients with dementia tends to get overwhelming, especially when one person is handling every task pertaining to the patient's care. This involves both mental and physical help, along with managing appointments, ensuring proper administration of medications, and taking care of the patient's schedule, including their meal time, workout timing, and sleep cycle. When two or more people come forward to share these responsibilities, the chances of the situation getting overwhelmingly tiring are reduced drastically, and the duties are managed rather smoothly and more efficiently.

Better Decision-Making

When one person has to make all the decisions pertaining to the health of a patient with dementia, it serves not only as a huge responsibility but also makes decision-making a difficult process because of limited ideas. In the case of a team of caregivers, this process becomes easier and much smoother, providing multiple ideas so that the best decision can be made with regard to the patient's health. Also, it allows caregivers to share the responsibility of making decisions for the patient without one person having to deal with responsibility as uncompromisingly significant as deciding what's best for the patient.

Professional, Specialized Care

It does not always have to be a family member, and there is nothing wrong with it. Patients with dementia can be taken care of by a team of professionals who are equipped with specialized skills and trained in dealing with everything pertaining to the patient. Whether it comes to administering a patient's medications, providing meals as per a well-designed schedule, bathing the patient, taking the patient for a stroll, or providing the patient with therapy for both physical and mental health, a team of trained professionals can prove to more fruitful than the patient being under the care of a family member. While nothing matches the sincerity and love rooted in bonds of blood, a team of professional caregivers can prove to be incredibly advantageous, given that each member of the team would be a master of their own specified task. As a result, patients with dementia can get thorough, specialized care.

Improved Flow of Communication

Communication plays a vital role in providing thorough care and support for those who struggle to live their lives due to chronic conditions such as dementia. When people team up to provide care and assistance to patients with dementia, it becomes essential for these individuals to have channels of communication that ensure the right information is shared from one end to another. Regular communication keeps everyone informed about the patient's condition, any changes to treatment, and caregiving responsibilities in a collaborative caregiving paradigm. Caretakers stay organized and in sync when they use common resources like calendars, apps, or group chats, which facilitates caregiving and reduces conflict.

The Takeaway

Caregiving is an essential tool for making life bearable for patients who develop dementia and diseases that fall under it. When one person takes on the responsibility of looking after a patient with dementia, there are many places when that one person can feel overwhelmed with a sense of losing control over the situation. Also, being constantly available for someone to provide mental and physical as well as emotional support is highly likely to make you feel drained. As a result, you may not be able to do a sufficient job, let alone an incredible one, when taking care of a patient with dementia. Besides, you may end up getting sick yourself. You can experience a decline in your physical and mental health. You can reach burnout earlier than usual, and you may end up finding yourself drifting into the abyss of mental issues.

Having someone to share your responsibilities with is not only beneficial for the one being taken care of but also for you.

Collaborative caregiving allows you to share your burden with those who collaborate with you to make the living experience better for the patients who have dementia. A collective endeavor ensures the well-being of not just the one who is ill but also the one who is looking after the patient.

Part VI:
Legal and Financial Essentials

Chapter 16: A Legal Framework for Elder Care

In order to provide seniors and their families with security, clarity, and peace of mind, legal preparations are a key factor in elder care. As people age, they may experience cognitive and physical impairments that make it challenging for them to handle their personal affairs, healthcare, and finances independently. Appropriate legal documents guarantee that their desires are respected and that they get the safety and care they require as they age. And cognitive impairments that hinder their ability to handle their personal affairs, healthcare, and finances effectively. As they age, legal documents guarantee that their desires are honored and that they get the safety and care they require.

There are some key reasons as to why legal preparations are essential when it comes to placing elders in care. They are enlisted below.

Upholding the Elder's Desires

Making legal arrangements guarantees that an older adult's wishes about their health, finances, and final care are accurately recorded and honored. Seniors can specify their preferences for medical care, inheritance, and other important decisions by creating important papers such as living wills, advance directives, and wills. In the absence of these records, the elder's desires can be disregarded, resulting in choices that go against their preferences.

Avoiding Family Disagreements

Caring for an elderly family member can be challenging since it calls for making several tough decisions, particularly in cases where there are no legal directives. Legal preparations help avoid conflicts by setting out procedures that every family member agrees to follow. For instance, a will or trust that has been properly drafted indicates the ways in which inheritance is to be distributed, thereby averting potential disputes. Assigning a durable power of attorney assures that a named suitable person can make decisions concerning the elder in their absence thus diminishing the chances for disputes within the family members concerned.

Protecting the Assets of the Elderly

As the age catches up with people, the task of saving money generally becomes tricky. In older Americans, unlike trusts against spending the proceeds with the call or money managing powers, carefully designed entities are put in place to care for the stuck or elders. Proper legal planning can assist victims in avoiding or eliminating possible financial exploitation and ease the responsible agents in ensuring that the caring funds are appropriate. Long-term care insurance, trusts, and estate planning in general are also capable of transferring the tax burden and ensuring the protection of resources from being exhausted by the expenses of long-term care services.

Securing Against Incapacity

A number of older adults are able to make legal preparations which ensures there are appointed representatives who are able to make decisions on their behalf when they are no longer truthful to their own affairs. With the formation of an advance health directive and a durable power of attorney it's possible to appoint a trusted agent able to make decisions in the event an elder is incapacitated. In these circumstances, the legal authority that's provided can be useful for an elder who suffers from any cognitive impairment or is unable to run their own affairs.

Facilitating the Making of Medical Care Related Decisions

End-of-life care and life support equipment and procedures involve an elder's legal agent making definitive decisions that may be difficult or involve the chances of feeling emotionally lost and confused. It makes it easier for them to choose between resuscitation, life support, a living will, or a healthcare proxy. The legal documentation assists the elder, the health care providers, and the family members to avoid any painful and, in certain moments, confusing and delaying situations by ensuring the elder's medical services are rendered according to their expressed wishes.

Avoiding Probate Courts and Legal Taxes

One of the legal services for seniors, especially estate planning, is the preparation of legal documents that allow one to avoid probate, which can be a long and expensive legal procedure if the person is deceased without having made a will or prepared legal documents. The establishment of trusts or wills is the way in which families could help mitigate the time and expense incurred in probate. More so, legal preparations can cut down estate taxes, thus ensuring that there are more assets left to the heirs instead of wasting on legal fees or taxes.

Obtaining Their Target:

Legal preparations regarding elder care have a significant amount of weight, and so do the reasons regarding this care, but the most weighty percentage of them is because of the peace of mind they offer. Seniors are going to be calm, knowing that their affairs have been handled well and that their intentions will be respected. Families will have these legal documents and, therefore, will not be pressed in difficult situations where such decisions are needed, and no aid is available. Legal preparations lessen the ambiguity and provide a sense of comfort during difficult times.

Comprehending Estate Planning

Estate planning can seem hard, but it is really about making sure that what your loved ones want is done when they can no longer say it. For older adults, estate planning keeps their belongings safe, secures their finances, and gives them and their families a sense of relief. Estate planning is not only for rich people—anyone who has belongings or specific desires about their healthcare or how their belongings should be shared should create a plan.

This includes writing a will, creating trusts, selecting healthcare agents, and giving power of attorney. The aim of estate planning is to stop avoidable legal and financial hassles after someone passes away or cannot make decisions. Having clear, legal documents can help avoid fights and make sure family members and healthcare workers can act on what the elder want. A good estate plan should address these questions:

Who gets the property or belongings?

Deciding who will inherit a person's property or assets upon their death is one of the most important things in estate planning. Without a clear plan, disagreements over the division of property can arise among family members, leading to disputes and lengthy legal battles. Writing a will is an important step in the process, allowing an individual to express their wishes and designate the beneficiaries of their assets—from property priorities to financial assets.

However, it's more than just supporting wishes; it's important to discuss these decisions with your loved ones to avoid potential misunderstandings. Consider hiring an estate planning attorney who can provide guidance on the various laws surrounding inheritance. Additionally, trust structures may be considered as they provide greater control over how and when assets are distributed. Ultimately, clear and careful planning allows people to manage their assets according to their wishes, giving themselves and their families peace of mind.

Who decides on healthcare or financial matters if the senior cannot?

When seniors are no longer able to make suitable decisions about their health or financial matters, it becomes important to choose a guardian. Designating a power of attorney (POA) is one good way to ensure that a trusted person can step in. A health care proxy allows a person to appoint someone to make medical decisions on their behalf if they become incapacitated. Similarly, a financial responsibility attorney allows a trusted individual to handle financial matters, ensure bills are paid, and manage the business.

These arrangements not only provide clarity but also prevent conflicts that can arise between family members. Seniors should discuss their options with potential decision-makers and clearly document their goals so everyone is on the same page. It is also important to review these documents regularly, as a person's circumstances can change over time. Carefully answering the question of who is responsible for making important decisions can ensure that seniors receive the care and financial management they need without placing an unnecessary burden on their families.

How will taxes or debts be managed after death?

Managing taxes and debts after a person's death can be a stressful experience for family members. It is important to note that the deceased's estate is usually responsible for any outstanding debts, meaning that creditors must be paid before the estate can be distributed to the heirs. This process begins with identifying all assets and liabilities, and involves the involvement of a lawyer or financial advisor to navigate the complex tax implications. For example, the estate may be required to file a final tax return showing all income up to the date of death.

More so, there are certain thresholds and liabilities for inheritance tax, which can have a significant impact on the amount of money left to the heirs. Importantly, clear records and arrangements can alleviate this burden, as all financial documents can be easily managed in the estate. Families should also consider discussing their estate planning options with a financial planner to ensure that taxes and debts are handled efficiently, minimizing stress during difficult times. Ultimately, knowledge and preparation can go a long way in addressing these issues, thereby preserving the legacy that society wants to leave behind.

Estate planning involves more than just the basics; it involves making difficult and critical decisions to protect the future of your loved ones. This also helps to avoid conflicts that can arise in a family when there is no legal documentation. Let's understand this by looking at something that provides a basic idea of it all: the will.

How to Draft a Will

A will is a fundamental part of estate planning. It's a legal document that specifies how a person's assets will be distributed after their death. For seniors, drafting a will is crucial to ensure that their property is passed on to the right individuals and that their final wishes are honored.

The Basics of a Will

A will should clearly state who the senior wishes to inherit their assets, designate an executor (the individual responsible for executing the will's terms), and include any specific instructions regarding the distribution of property. For instance, a grandparent might want to bequeath certain family heirlooms to a specific grandchild or allocate a portion of their estate to a charitable organization.

How to Get Started:

List All Assets: Start by compiling a comprehensive list of all assets, such as real estate, savings, retirement accounts, and personal belongings.

Identify Beneficiaries: These are the individuals who will inherit the assets. Beneficiaries can include family members, friends, or organizations like charities.

Name an Executor: The executor is responsible for ensuring that the will's terms are fulfilled. This person should be trustworthy and capable of managing financial and legal responsibilities.

Legal Requirements for a Will

Each state has its own regulations regarding what constitutes a legally binding will. Typically, a will needs to be signed in the presence of witnesses, who must also sign the document. It's wise to consult with an attorney to make sure the will adheres to state laws and addresses any potential issues that may arise.

Updating a Will

As life circumstances evolve, it's crucial to periodically review and update a will. For instance, if a senior undergoes a significant life change—like the birth of a grandchild, the passing of a spouse, or the sale of a property—the will should be revised to reflect these new developments.

Trusts: Options or Additions to Wills

Although wills are important, they are not sufficient to cover complex financial situations or to transfer assets. This is where trust comes in. A trust is a legal arrangement that allows one person (the trustee) to hold property for another person (the beneficiary). Trusts can be an effective way to manage assets, reduce estate taxes, and ensure that assets are distributed after death without the need for probate - a legal requirement in preparing a will.

Types of Trusts

There are several types of trusts that seniors and their families can consider. The trustee can modify or revoke a trust at any time. When the grantor dies, the assets are transferred to the beneficiaries without probate. This type of trust is ideal for those who want flexibility and want to avoid the delays associated with probate.

Irrevocable Trust:

Unlike a revocable trust, it cannot be easily changed once it is created. This type of trust removes assets from the grantor's taxable estate, which can be useful for reducing estate taxes. However, the lender must have control of the property.

Special Care:

This is designed for beneficiaries who are disabled or require long-term care. A special needs trust can use assets for the care of the beneficiary without affecting their eligibility for government assistance programs such as Medicaid.

Charitable Trust:

For those who want to leave a portion of their estate to charity, a charitable trust is a good option. This trust can provide tax benefits and support essential services for the individual.

Advantages of a Trust

A trust has several advantages over a will, especially when it comes to managing assets and providing protection for beneficiaries. Here are some of the advantages of setting up a trustee:

Avoiding Probate:

One important advantage of a trust is its ability to bypass a time-consuming and expensive process. Unlike a will, which must go through probate court, a trust allows assets to be transferred directly to beneficiaries, saving time and legal costs. This allows the space to be efficiently and quickly arranged.

Privacy:

When a will passes the test, it becomes part of a public registry, meaning that anyone can access information about assets and their distribution.

Trusts, in disparity, are private. The purposes of a trust, including the distribution of assets and beneficiaries, are not publicly disclosed, ensuring the privacy and discretion of the family.

Ongoing management:

Trusts provide great flexibility and control over the distribution of assets. They can be designed to distribute assets in installments rather than all at once.

This can be especially beneficial for young beneficiaries or those who need financial guidance, as the trust can gradually meet their needs and provide financial stability.

Protection for beneficiaries:

A trust can provide protection for the beneficiary by shielding assets from creditors or legal claims, which is especially useful if the beneficiary is financially unstable or in danger.

Trustees also allow for conditions to be set about when and how the beneficiaries receive the assets, adding additional security.

Ability to act on changes:

A trust can be amended or modified when circumstances change, for example, changes in the beneficiaries' needs or new legal changes. This flexibility allows for great flexibility in landscaping.

These advantages make trusts attractive to those who want a safe, efficient, and private way to manage and distribute their assets.

Power of Attorney: Managing Financial and Healthcare Decisions

As people age, it can become increasingly difficult to manage their finances or make healthcare decisions due to illness or decreased understanding. That's why a power of attorney (POA) is important. A POA is a legal document that gives a trustee the authority to make financial or medical decisions on behalf of another person.

Types of Powers of Attorney

Powers of attorney are important legal documents that give one person the authority to make decisions on behalf of another person. There are several types of power of attorney, each of which serves different purposes, especially when it comes to managing financial, legal, and health care decisions for older adults. Here are the main types of authorization:

General Power of Attorney:

This document gives broad authority to manage financial matters, including paying bills, signing checks, managing investments, and managing property. However, it can be inconvenient if the person becomes incapacitated.

Durable Power of Attorney:

Unlike a regular POA, a durable power of attorney remains in effect even if the person becomes incapacitated. This is especially important for seniors who are at risk of mental illness. A durable power of attorney allows an attorney-in-fact to be appointed to manage the senior's finances, ensure their debts are paid, and effectively manage their assets.

Health Care Power of Attorney:

This gives the trustee the authority to make health care decisions when the senior is unable to do so. It is important for seniors to choose someone who understands their healthcare preferences and can support them when needed.

Guardianship: When Legal Permission Is Needed

At times, an elder may be unable to make decisions for himself because of a troubled conscience, illness, or physical infirmity. Without proper legal documentation, such as power of attorney or advance directives, so that others can help them, families face a great deal of stress and burden. When this happens, families have no choice but to seek legal guardianship or custody through the courts.

The process of obtaining legal counsel involves asking the court to appoint someone to make decisions for the elder, including matters related to health care, housing, and finances. This procedure is necessary when previous legal authority is lost, and the elderly are no longer able to make reasonable decisions on their own. The Inspectorate provides legal authority to the client, allowing a designated inspector to review the decision if they wish.

However, the work can be tiring for the family. There will be an opportunity to prove the officer's incompetence through medical evaluation and evidence, but this may not be possible and may lead to family disputes or conflicts. In addition, the court must carefully review the legality of the proposed guardian to ensure that he or she is acting in the interests of the principal and has the authority to perform the tasks. In some cases, if family members cannot agree on a guardian, or there are no suitable relatives, the court can appoint a person with political rights and duties.

While guardianship provides legal authority to protect a senior's health, safety, and property, seniors also retain their own autonomy. Therefore, administrative jurisdiction should be considered a last resort unless other legal tools (such as power of attorney or a health care provider) have been established in advance.

Bottomline

Legal planning for elder care is not about managing assets but about protecting rights, respecting your wishes, and providing emotional support for the elderly and their families. By following the steps to create a will, trust, power of attorney and advance directive, seniors can plan for their future and reduce the legal worries of their loved ones.

Early preparation is important. By starting legal planning discussions early, families can ensure their loved ones are cared for according to their wishes while minimizing legal hassles and complications.

The legal implications described in this chapter can make caring for an older adult easier and more compassionate for everyone. By addressing these challenges, families can face the challenges of aging with confidence, knowing their loved ones are protected and their wishes are respected.

Chapter 17: Planning for the Financial Realities

Taking care of an elderly who suffers from conditions like Alzheimer's and Parkinson's disease is no easy feat. It requires a great deal of patience and more than that, it requires resources. Arranging those resources comes with a lot of challenges. Those challenges can be financial binds as well as emotional tolls, which may not allow the caregiver to breathe an air of peace and calm. However, if the caregiver has the right set of tips and techniques, both financial challenges and emotional issues can be well be taken care of. But for that to be taken care of, one needs to know what problems one is likely to face when one chooses to take responsibility, as huge as taking care of an elderly whose mental health deteriorates every passing moment of the day.

There is no doubt that there is going to be a plethora of problems. But a wise man once said that a problem written is a problem half-solved. Listing down the problems you are most likely to have when you take up such responsibility will help you in ways unimaginable. However, you will only be able to list those problems down once you know what those problems could be. Some of those issues you may not even know that you are likely to encounter. Therefore, to help you navigate through those problems, this chapter aims to highlight potential issues a caregiver is likely to encounter once the caregiver starts taking care of the elderly suffering from dementia and diseases that fall under the canopy of dementia.

There's More to the List Than You Know

Life is not the same for everyone. While many of us don't have to fend for others other than ourselves, it's different for many. For several families, elder care is an unavoidable stage of life that presents both financial and emotional difficulties. Families must make tough choices about how to give their loved ones the greatest care possible as they get older. The financial strain of elder care is an unavoidable truth, even though emotional factors frequently take priority. Elder care can be quite expensive, and families frequently have to change their budgets, take money out of savings, or negotiate a confusing web of payment alternatives and government aid programs. Financial planning is a crucial component of elder care since these costs can affect not only the elderly individuals but also their families.

The Cost that Comes with Taking Care of the Elderly

The cost of providing elder care frequently begins gradually and rises over time. Many older adults start out with only basic help, including assistance with cooking or cleaning. But as people age, they may require more extensive care, such as medical support, personal care services, and perhaps full-time residential care. Every one of these phases entails additional expenses, which can mount up rapidly. Families frequently experience financial stress and struggle to make decisions because they are ill-prepared for the high costs of assisted living facilities, nursing homes, and in-home care.

The typical expense of long-term care in a nursing home can surpass $100,000 per year in the United States alone. The monthly expense of even less intensive forms of care, like adult daycare or home health aides, can reach thousands of dollars. Many families are shocked to hear that many of these expenses may not be covered by Medicare and standard health insurance, forcing them to rely on private insurance, personal savings, or government programs like Medicaid, each of which has its own restrictions and requirements.

Financial Hardships and Management

Managing elder care costs is complicated in ways that go beyond the actual costs. It cannot be easy to navigate the several government programs, commercial funding choices, and payment options. In addition to attempting to manage the emotional strain of caring for a loved one, families must interpret complicated legislation and foreign terminology. Medicaid, for instance, can be a lifeline for many families, but qualifying frequently necessitates careful planning or major changes in a family's financial circumstances, and eligibility is determined by stringent financial requirements. Funding can also be obtained through long-term care insurance or reverse mortgages, but each option has advantages and disadvantages that should be carefully considered.

The financial difficulties associated with elder care can also last for years or even decades, making it a long-term commitment. Because of this fact, early financial preparation is only beneficial. Many people assume that savings or health insurance would cover the costs of elder care, so they don't properly plan for it. Families may, however, find it difficult to make ends meet while giving the required care if they are unaware of the full costs and the options that are accessible. Families navigating elder care can have a simpler journey by preparing ahead of time, considering all of their alternatives, and getting financial counsel as soon as possible.

Financial hardship frequently exacerbates the emotional and physical toll of caregiving, resulting in a complex burden that can affect relationships and individual well-being. In addition to having their own financial obligations, such as providing for their own children or saving for retirement, adult children are sometimes entrusted with making financial decisions for their elderly parents. Without the right assistance and planning, juggling the demands of caring for others, handling money, and making future plans might become too much to handle.

Such and many other financial factors and difficulties related to elder care will be addressed in the text subsequential in this chapter. Exploring thoroughly the financial aspect of caregiving, from comprehending the significant range in costs to determining the elements that impact them, some key aspects of taking care of older adults through financial means will also be mentioned. You will have a better grasp of how to handle the financial aspects of elder care by the end of this chapter, which will help you make sure your loved ones get the care they need without endangering the financial security of your family.

It's Not Limited to Just Emotions

To be precise, the financial element of caregiving is just as important as the emotional and practical components, which frequently take center stage. Families may make well-informed decisions, lessen stress, and concentrate on what really matters—giving their loved ones high-quality care in their later years—if they have the necessary information and preparation.

The financial landscape of elder care is as complex as it is varied. No two families face the same set of circumstances, and the cost of elder care can differ dramatically based on the type of care needed, the region in which it is provided, and the duration of care required. For many families, the journey begins with minimal support, such as occasional in-home assistance or respite care. It may progress over time to more intensive forms of care, like assisted living or nursing home residency. This variability in costs is not just about numbers—it represents the reality of the aging process, which is unpredictable and often comes with difficult choices that pull at both heartstrings and wallets.

One key factor influencing elder care costs is the setting in which care is provided. For individuals who can continue living at home, initial expenses may be relatively manageable. Home care services, such as part-time assistance with daily activities, typically range from $20 to $40 per hour, depending on the level of support needed and the geographic location. This can be a practical solution for families requiring only a few hours of help each week.

Things Change Over the Course of Time

However, as a loved one's needs evolve, it's essential to be prepared for potential increases in costs. If around-the-clock care becomes necessary, families may face significantly higher expenses. Being proactive about planning and exploring various care options can help manage these costs effectively. Families can benefit from seeking resources and support networks to navigate the challenges of caregiving while maintaining the regular expenses associated with home upkeep.

Take the case of Alice, whose 82-year-old father, Robert, was initially able to live independently with only minor assistance. Alice hired a part-time caregiver to visit him twice a week for a few hours to help with meals and light housework, costing her roughly $500 per month. However, over the course of two years, Robert's health deteriorated, and he began to need more frequent help. His caregiver started visiting daily, assisting with bathing, dressing, and medication management. Soon, Alice found herself spending $4,000 a month just to keep her father at home, and the emotional toll of managing his care alongside her own career and family responsibilities became overwhelming. While this may be a hypothetical situation, this is not entirely far from reality.

Home care can seem like the greatest choice for families like Alice's since it keeps their loved ones in familiar settings while preserving their independence and dignity. The emotional advantages of in-home care must eventually be weighed against the rising expenses, though, as the financial load frequently grows over time. At this point, many families start looking at alternative elder care options, such as nursing homes or assisted living facilities, each of which has its own set of financial difficulties.

When Living Requires Assistance

Assisted living is a prevalent choice for those who require more support than in-home care can provide but do not yet need the level of medical care offered in nursing homes. Assisted living facilities offer a more structured environment, with staff available to assist residents with daily activities, medication management, and meal preparation while still allowing for some level of independence. However, this support comes at a significant cost. Depending on location, the average monthly cost of an assisted living facility in the U.S. ranges from $4,000 to $7,000, with some high-end facilities charging even more for additional services or luxury amenities. This monthly expense can quickly add up, making assisted living unaffordable for many families without careful financial planning.

Think about Tom and his wife, Judith, who were forced to relocate into an assisted living facility when Judith's Parkinson's disease made it impossible for her to do everyday chores by herself. The pair initially valued the facility's social events and sense of community, and they were relieved to have access to round-the-clock help. But within a year, their assisted living bills had risen to $90,000, which was significantly more than they had anticipated. Even though Judith received first-rate care, Tom had to take money out of their retirement account to pay for it, which made him concerned about his own financial future. The example of Tom and Judith being yet another hypothetical situation. Their circumstances are similar to many people going through the same ordeal.

Nursing Homes — a Better Option?

For those who require more intensive, medical-based care, nursing homes represent the highest tier of elder care. Nursing homes provide around-the-clock skilled nursing care and are equipped to handle complex medical needs, making them a necessary option for those suffering from severe health conditions, such as advanced dementia or debilitating chronic illnesses. However, this level of care comes with a price. In the U.S., the average annual cost of a private room in a nursing home exceeds $100,000, with costs varying significantly depending on the location and quality of the facility. For many families, this expense is simply unaffordable without government assistance or private long-term care insurance.

Deciding to move a loved one into a nursing home is often filled with emotional and financial challenges. Nursing homes, especially those that specialize in memory care or skilled nursing, can be quite expensive. Families need to consider not only the quality of care provided but also the financial implications of this decision. The average annual cost of nursing home care exceeds $100,000, which can deplete personal savings or retirement funds, putting families in a difficult financial situation. Furthermore, nursing homes may have unexpected or hidden costs, including fees for specific medical services, personal care, and even recreational activities for residents.

Some families can afford nursing home care through a mix of personal savings and long-term care insurance. However, others must look for alternative funding options. For many, government programs like Medicaid are crucial for covering these costs, but accessing Medicaid often requires families to meet strict financial criteria. This may involve spending down assets or restructuring finances in ways that can feel overwhelming or unfair. The complexities of Medicaid eligibility add to the stress of an already challenging decision, forcing families to make significant sacrifices to ensure their loved ones receive the necessary care.

Professional Guidance

It's important for families to understand the eligibility requirements for Medicaid, which may involve restructuring finances or spending down assets. While this process can seem daunting, there are resources and specialists who can help guide families through the complexities of financial planning for long-term care. Ultimately, with informed decision-making and a proactive approach, families can ensure their loved ones receive the care they need while managing the financial implications effectively.

Variability of Cost

The variability in elder care costs is significantly influenced by geographic factors. In general, elder care is more expensive in urban areas than in rural ones, primarily due to higher wages, property costs, and greater demand for services. For instance, the cost of elder care in major metropolitan areas like New York City or San Francisco can be nearly double that of similar services in smaller towns or rural regions. This geographic disparity can create challenges for families in deciding where their loved ones will receive care. It may lead them to consider relocating their relatives to areas with lower costs, even if these places are farther away from family members who provide emotional support.

Ultimately, the wide range of elder care costs reflects the diversity of needs and circumstances faced by aging individuals and their families. There is no one-size-fits-all solution, and each family must carefully weigh their options, considering both the emotional and financial implications of their decisions.

Factors Affecting the Cost of Taking Care of Elders

When evaluating the costs associated with elder care, it's crucial to recognize the various key factors that significantly impact expenses. By understanding these components, families can make informed decisions and choose the best care options for their loved ones, ensuring their comfort and well-being.

Here are a few pointers that show what factors affect the cost of taking care of the elders:

The Location:

Cost of Living: Urban areas generally have a higher cost of living, which directly affects the pricing of elder care services, including housing and staffing.

Availability of Services: Urban areas often offer a wider variety of care facilities. However, increased competition does not always lead to lower costs. In contrast, rural areas may have fewer options but tend to offer more affordable rates.

Travel Costs: In rural regions, the costs associated with transportation to medical facilities can be significant, especially when specialized care is required.

Staffing Costs: Urban centers typically need to pay higher wages for care staff, which contributes to the overall cost of elder care services.

Different Levels of Care Needed:

Basic Assistance: Individuals who only need help with daily activities, such as bathing and dressing, usually pay less than those who require full-time medical supervision.

Medical Needs: Patients with chronic illnesses or conditions like dementia need specialized care, which significantly increases costs.

Skilled Nursing: Those who require regular medical care, such as wound management or medication administration, will face higher costs for trained professionals.

Memory Care Units: Facilities designed for patients with Alzheimer's or other memory-related conditions are more expensive due to the need for specialized staff and secure environments.

Physical Therapy and Rehabilitation: After surgery or for mobility-related issues, physical therapy may be required, which adds another layer of expense.

Dedicated Services:

Personalized Care Plans: Some facilities provide individualized care plans. While these plans can be beneficial, they may be more expensive than standardized packages.

Special Dietary Needs: Facilities that accommodate specific diets (such as diabetic or gluten-free) may charge additional fees for customized meal preparation.

Transportation for Appointments: Care facilities that offer transportation to medical appointments might have extra charges for these services.

On-site Medical Staff: Access to doctors or nurses within the care facility can increase costs, especially in high-demand areas.

Recreational Activities: Engaging in social activities, such as art classes, outings, and fitness programs, can also contribute to the overall cost of elder care.

By identifying these essential factors, families can more effectively anticipate elder care expenses and make informed financial decisions to meet their loved one's needs.

Tactics for Having Enough Money for Elder Care

Although elder care can be very expensive, families can better control these costs with careful preparation and calculated methods. Individuals can lessen financial stress and guarantee that their loved ones receive the care they require by combining a variety of strategies, such as budgeting, investigating insurance alternatives, and consulting a specialist. The following are some useful strategies for managing elder care expenses:

1. Creating a Comprehensive Budget

There's always a solution for every problem, budget being one of them. We tend to come across challenges and financial difficulties because, more often than not, we do not plan our expenses. We may have a budget, but can we be sure that the budget we drafted was enough? Does that budget cover every minor to major expense that we are likely to incur? It is, therefore, quite necessary to have a budget that covers everything precisely. To be able to deal with the financial challenges that come with taking care of people who have dementia, we need a comprehensive budget that covers every single expense that we are *likely* to incur.

Unearth Current Expenses: Dive deep into the world of elder care costs! Identify every penny spent on home modifications, caregiving services, medical supplies, and transportation to paint a complete picture of your financial landscape.

Anticipate Future Needs: Life is unpredictable, especially when it comes to care requirements. Think ahead and prepare for potential shifts, such as moving from occasional assistance to full-time care or making the leap to an assisted living community.

Embrace Inflation: Keep in mind that the costs of care services don't stay stagnant—they tend to rise over time. Factor in inflation to your long-term care budget to stay ahead of the curve and avoid surprises.

Identify What Matters Most: Create a hierarchy of needs by ranking your most critical expenses. Focus on the essentials—like medical care and personal assistance—to ensure that your top priorities are taken care of first.

Stay on Top of Spending: Take control of your financial journey by using budgeting apps or financial tools. Keep a close eye on ongoing elder care costs and be ready to make adjustments along the way. Remember, proactive tracking is key to a secure financial future!

Explore Your Insurance Choices

Navigating the world of elder care can be overwhelming, but exploring your insurance options can offer peace of mind and financial relief.

Long-Term Care Insurance: Investing in a long-term care insurance policy can provide coverage for a variety of essential services, from home health care to assisted living and nursing homes. The key is to act early—premiums tend to increase as we age, so the sooner you start, the better!

Health Insurance and Medicare: Get to know your traditional health insurance and Medicare coverage limits. While Medicare does a great job covering short-term rehabilitation and hospital stays, it typically falls short for long-term care services.

Medicare Advantage Plans: Consider investigating Medicare Advantage plans; some of these may provide limited coverage for in-home care or other services that standard Medicare overlooks. This could mean less out-of-pocket spending for you!

Hybrid Life Insurance Policies: Think about hybrid life insurance options that include long-term care riders. These smart policies let you tap into funds for elder care if the need arises, all while securing your family's financial future.

Veterans' Benefits: If you or your spouse is a veteran, don't forget to check into potential long-term care benefits through the Department of Veterans Affairs. These special programs can significantly lighten your financial load when it comes to elder care.

By proactively exploring these options, you can ensure that you and your loved ones are well-prepared for future care needs.

3. Consider Housing and Living Arrangements

Making smart decisions about where a loved one will live can greatly affect elder care costs.

- **Home Modifications:** If your loved one can remain at home with some assistance, consider making home modifications, such as adding safety bars, stair lifts, or wheelchair ramps, to accommodate their needs. These one-time investments are often more affordable than moving into a facility.

- **Downsizing or Relocating:** If maintaining a large home is no longer practical, downsizing or relocating to a smaller, more manageable living space can save money on utilities, upkeep, and property taxes.

- **Shared Living Arrangements:** Consider shared living situations, such as moving an aging parent in with family members or opting for a senior co-housing arrangement where multiple individuals share the cost of care and housing.

4. Seek Professional Financial Advice

Navigating the financial landscape of elder care can be complex, so consulting with professionals who specialize in elder care planning is often a wise investment.

Hire a Financial Advisor: A financial advisor with expertise in elder care can help develop a long-term strategy to manage costs. They can also assist in assessing available assets, retirement accounts, and insurance policies.

Elder Care Planners: Eldercare planners are professionals who can guide families through the various options available for financing elder care. They can also assist in applying for benefits, such as Medicaid, and help families navigate eligibility requirements.

Tax Planning: Elder care costs can come with certain tax deductions, such as medical expenses or caregiver expenses. A tax professional can help identify deductions and credits that could reduce the overall tax burden associated with elder care.

The Takeaway

Elder care can appear to be a financial headache, especially when the elderly suffer from a condition like dementia. However, with the right planning and tools, families can make good decisions and come up with a good financial plan. You can also avoid financial stress in the future and be able to focus on giving quality care to your loved ones by being careful with your budget, looking into insurance, making the right housing decisions, and seeking professional help. You can reduce your financial stress and focus on quality care for your loved ones by planning wisely.

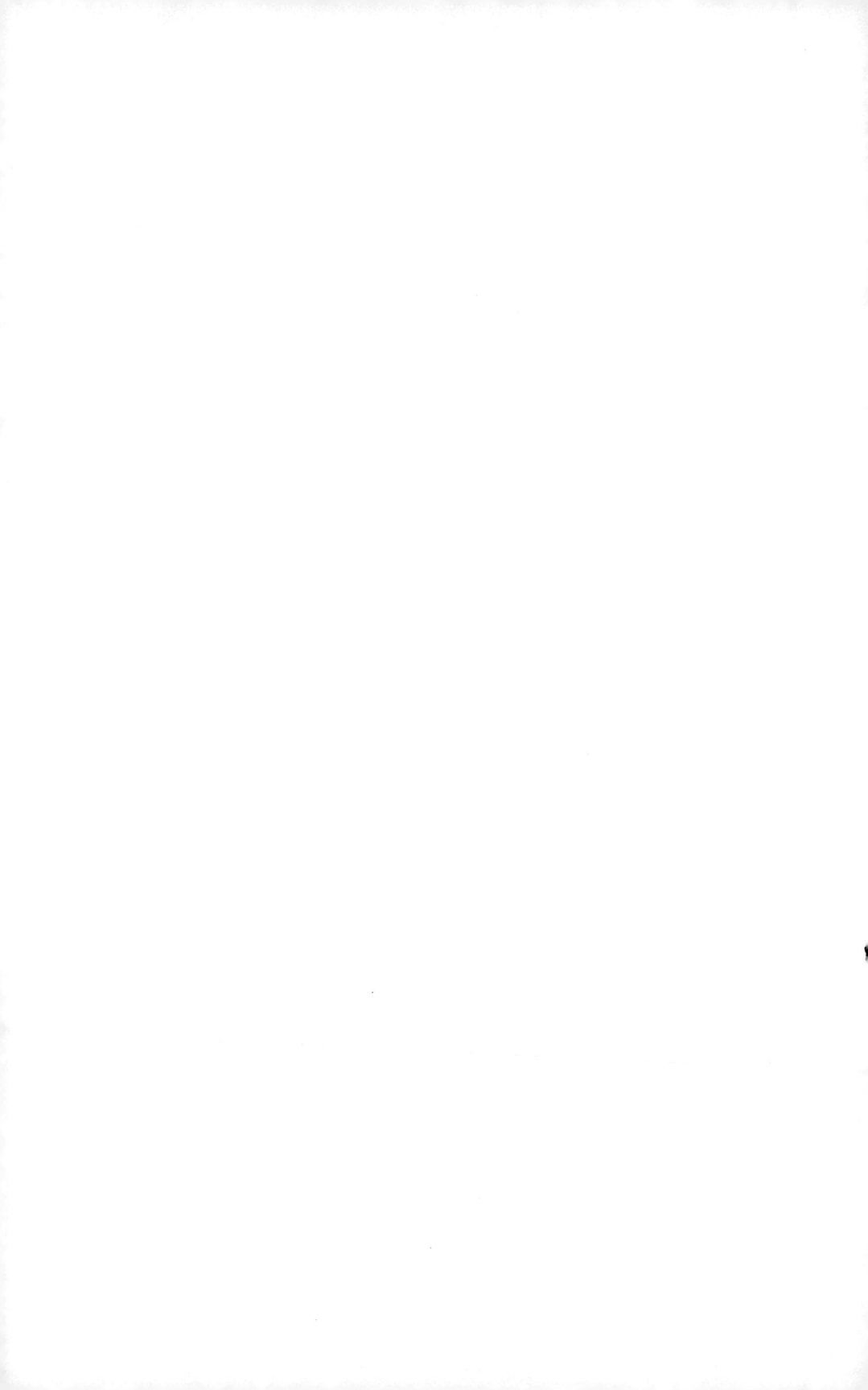

www.ingramcontent.com/pod-product-compliance
Lightning Source LLC
Chambersburg PA
CBHW052110030426
42335CB00025B/2918